MICHIGAN BUSINESS PAPERS

Number 60

The Department of Economics of Western Michigan University is pleased to cooperate with the Division of Research at the Graduate School of Business Administration, The University of Michigan, in presenting this collection of papers, in which six distinguished economists discuss economic aspects of U.S. public policy on medical care, present and proposed. This volume is the ninth in a series being published under these auspices.

MICHIGAN BUSINESS
PAPERS   Number 60

The U.S. Medical Care Industry:

The Economist's Point of View

*Six lectures on economic aspects of the medical
care system in the United States, given at Western
Michigan University under the sponsorship of the
Department of Economics, Winter 1974*

JOSEPH C. MORREALE, Editor

A publication of the
Division of Research
Graduate School of Business Administration
University of Michigan
Ann Arbor, Michigan

ISBN-0-87712-166-4

Copyright © 1974

by

The University of Michigan

To
Betty
Gwen and Meg

CONTENTS

PREFACE

The two main concepts that economists are associated with in this analysis of real world problems are supply and demand, and these two concepts get translated into policy questions concerning efficiency and equity respectively. It should not be surprising, therefore, that when six distinguished economists take part in a lecture series dealing with the economics of health care the point of view taken centers around these two key concepts and these two key questions. However, this is not to say that these six economists all have the same point of view. In fact, you will see that their perspectives about the U.S. medical care system cover a fairly wide spectrum.

There has been much criticism of the U.S. medical care system from many sources. And yet, many of its good aspects are ignored. Professor Harry Schwartz provides an interesting defense of American medicine because he feels that most of the criticism about the U.S. medical care system is not based on fact. He refutes four major criticisms leveled at American medicine: (1) that the medical care system is of poor quality, (2) that because of this poor system, the health of the American people is deficient, (3) that there is a drastic, overall shortage of physicians, and (4) that medical care is terribly expensive.

Professor Schwartz contends that when one compares the United States with other nations having similar socioeconomic and demographic characteristics (like the USSR), one finds that the usual indices of health status indicate that the U.S. population is healthier. Moreover, he points out that there has been tremendous technological advancement in U.S. medical care, and the quality and quantity of medical resources in the U.S. medical care system are the envy of the world. He also argues that the United States is increasing its supply of physicians at a rate which is faster than that of population growth, and that no evil monopoly force (like the AMA) is holding back the production of physicians. And finally, he points out that, since most people in the United States are covered by some type of hospital insurance and the federal government will enact, sometime in the near future, a national health insurance plan, the problem of the high cost of medical care will be alleviated.

Professor Kessel, in his lecture focusing on the role that the AMA plays in all aspects of the U.S. medical care system, draws a striking contrast to Professor Schwartz's point of view on two main points. He asserts that, through its control of the production of physicians, the AMA has been responsible for the doctor shortage in the United States. In addition, Professor Kessel believes that, instead of having the best medical care system in the world, the United States really just has the most expensive system.

Professor Kessel contends that the AMA achieved monopoly control over the supply of physicians by means of the Flexner report of 1910. He mentions four main effects of the implementation of this report: (1) medical education became more expensive and narrowly standardized; (2) a sharp reduction occurred in the number of medical schools and in the number of new medical graduates;(3) there was a sharp reduction in black, Jewish, and female physicians; and (4) there has been a large increase in the number of American students studying medicine abroad.

Professor Kessel disputes the AMA contention that its action was based on a desire to raise the quality of physicians and thereby increase the quality of medical care in the United States. He argues that improved quality has increased the price of physician services, which has deterred the poor from receiving adequate medical care. Moreover, he insists that the AMA has supported practices and conditions which reduce the quality of care, and of these he mentions six main ones: (1) discrimination in terms of race, creed, and color in admission to medical schools; (2) grandfather clauses for existing practitioners who graduated from inferior medical schools; (3) the lack of required periodic reexamination of practicing physicians; (4) intertwining politics with decisions which should be only based on quality; (5) making decisions about staff appointments to hospitals on the basis of factors other than quality; and (6) inhibiting the free flow of information about the quality of care.

Professor Kessel points out two additional AMA policies which have helped cause the price of medical care to be artificially high. First, the AMA's imposition of a rigid, high-cost medical curriculum on medical schools has increased the cost of producing physicians and inhibited experimentation and innovation in the training of physicians. Second, the AMA's opposition to forms of medical care delivery systems which differ from the fee-for-service system has greatly inhibited the search for, and experimentation with, the delivery of medical services.

While Professor Kessel's paper can be viewed as an analysis of the influence of private AMA policy on the U.S. medical care system, Professor Rosenthal analyzes the need for public policy in the health services sector and the role of research in developing this policy. He provides two main reasons for having a public health care policy. First, the consumption and utilization of medical services exhibit externalities. That is, there are external benefits accruing to society by the consumption of such services, and there are external costs imposed on the society in the absence of such utilization. Second, health care is viewed as a right of all citizens. So, society insists that a public policy be adopted to insure that this right in fact exists.

Professor Rosenthal states an important law of policy which is particularly relevant to the health care market: When a society is faced with conflicting goals, one goal must be sacrificed in order to achieve the other. Or, to put it another way, no single policy can achieve two competing goals. He astutely points out a fundamental dilemma in health care policy: the trade-off between high quality services and the availability of services. Professor Rosenthal feels that the former usually overrides the latter, and Professor Kessel's analysis provides clear evidence that this does, in fact, occur.

Professor Rosenthal sees the role of research in developing public policy as one of testing the assumptions and effectiveness of the policy and objectively identifying the costs and the benefits of various strategies. He argues that, in this process, the working of the medical system is better understood and various policy options are offered.

There have been two major policy proposals before Congress which have stirred much controversy: to establish a National Health Insurance plan (NHI) and to support development of Health Maintenance Organizations (HMO). The former is a demand strategy and is supposed to deal with the equity problem. The latter is a supply strategy and is supposed to help solve the efficiency problem. Since these two issues are in the forefront of public debate, most of the speakers addressed themselves to at least one of these two issues.

Professor Herbert Klarman provides a detailed analysis of the issues surrounding national health insurance. He surveys the past successes and failures of voluntary health insurance plans and the Medicare and Medicaid programs. The four main advantages that he mentions are: (1) that insurance plans have demonstrated the practicability of buying health services through third parties; (2) the burden of major illness has been alleviated for many people; (3) the use of medical services by low income people has increased; and (4) most providers of health services have prospered financially.

On the other hand, Professor Klarman sees three main disadvantages. First, insurance plans have caused a steady increase in hospital use. Second, the expansion of health insurance plans has caused sharp increases in medical care prices. And third, there has been little change in the institutional and behavioral aspects of the U.S. health service system.

Professor Klarman proposes five criteria for assessing a national health insurance plan: (1) universal enrollment, (2) a uniform package of benefits that is both broad and deep for all, (3) furtherance of the goal of a single system of medical care for all, (4) effective provision for provider reimbursement with a responsible and responsive increase of regulatory authority rooted in a free flow of information, and (5) ease of compliance by consumers with attention to the validation of their expectations from the insurance plan.

Professor Rosenthal raises some important questions about how effective NHI will be in solving the equity problem. He foresees a further increase in the price of medical care and in the cost of government programs due to the passage of NHI. Based on past government reaction to increased costs of medical programs, such increases will most probably result in increased deductibles, establishment of some co-insurance feature, and perhaps a redefinition of eligibility. Such changes would move the allocation of medical resources back to the market's allocation. Moreover, Professor Rosenthal sees the main benefit of NHI going to those persons already able to obtain medical care, whereas those outside the present medical care system would remain outside. Both of these results would defeat the purpose of NHI, i.e., reallocation of medical resources to the needy.

Professor Schwartz feels that most of the NHI plans proposed are too expensive and involve too much government intervention in the medical care system. He adamantly opposes the Kennedy plan because he feels it would lead to the socialization of U.S. medicine. Instead, Professor Schwartz favors a simple, low cost, catastrophic health insurance plan (like the Long-Ribicoff Bill) which would help defray the exorbitant medical costs which are most devastating to individual families.

Additional proposals were made by some of the speakers concerning demand-side policies. Professor Feldstein suggests that information on provider performance, quality, and prices should be provided to the consumer so that the consumer can make more rational decisions in the marketplace. Professor Rosenthal would like to see the federal government guarantee some minimum adequate level of health services for each person in the United States. He feels that such a proposal would bring more services to those people who are presently outside of the medical care system and thereby achieve the equity objective.

Professor Paul Feldstein focuses his lecture on the supply side, or the efficiency question, concerning the delivery of health care services. He sees the responsiveness of the supply of medical services to the increased demand for such services as crucial. In his view, the nature of the supply response will not only influence the cost of medical care but will also determine how effective and how large government programs for redistributing medical service will be. He points out various factors of the medical care market which have inhibited increases in supply and have fostered inefficiency in supply: cost reimbursement methods of paying hospitals, reasonable and customary fee methods of paying physicians, numerous barriers to entry in various health care professions, overemphasis on high quality training of health professionals, and prohibitions on competitive advertising by health professionals.

One particular policy on the supply side which is being widely discussed is the development of Health Maintenance Organizations (HMOs). An HMO is a prepaid group plan offering a comprehensive set of services to a particular group of contractors on a capitation payment basis. Professor Feldstein is very much in favor of a large-scale expansion of HMOs in the United States. He argues that an HMO has greater incentive to be efficient in the delivery of medical care, it will serve as a competitor to the fee-for-service system, and it is better able to relate the training requirements of personnel to the tasks to be performed. Professor Kessel favors the HMO idea because an HMO will be more able to reduce prices for surgical services, link the buying of surgical and nonsurgical services at prices that reflect their relative costs of production, and provide more information to the public about various aspects of medical care. Professor Klarman adds that an HMO will provide more free choice to the consumer, and Professor Rosenthal feels that an HMO's main advantage is cost containment.

On the other hand, there are some drawbacks to HMOs. Professor Schwartz argues that an HMO is more apt to be inefficient. He contends that when the fee-for-service is eliminated, the medical system is flooded by the "worried well" who "usurp" the medical resources available to treat the sick. Moreover, Professor Schwartz feels that when a price is not linked to a specific service, there is an incentive to waste resources.

Professor Klarman, though favoring their development, mentions certain concerns that he has with HMOs. He points out that the saving in hospital use by HMOs has not been unambiguously determined, and prepaid group practice has not generated extra productivity in the use of personnel. Moreover, Professors Klarman and Rosenthal feel that the present HMO Bill recently passed by the Congress does an injustice to HMOs. It requires HMOs to provide too broad a package of services and subjects HMOs to quality controls that apply to nobody else in the medical care system. In so doing, Congress tried to simultaneously achieve two conflicting goals, increased quantity and high quality, which is an impossibility. Professor Rosenthal predicts that Congress will be either forced to subvert the high standards that it has established or to increase the start-up money so that a subsidized, high quality HMO can be tried as a pilot project.

Professor Donald Yett's analysis of the market for nurses focuses on an interesting example of another type of federal government supply policy, in this case one specifically designed to increase the supply of nurses. The analysis also provides us with a good example of the role of research in policy making which Rosenthal emphasized.

At the prompting of the 1963 Report of the Surgeon General's Consulting Group on Nursing, which concluded that there would be a severe shortage of nurses by 1970, Congress initiated a large nurse-training subsidy program in 1964 (Nurse Training Act) and authorized the expenditure of $1.3 billion over the past decade. Professor Yett points out that the basic goal set down by the Consulting Group—to increase the total supply of nurses—was achieved by 1969, but the annual number of graduates from nursing schools only increased very slightly. These conflicting results raise the question: Was the Nurse Training Act (NTA) successful?

Professor Yett points out that, in order to maximize the benefit of a program designed to increase the supply of manpower via training subsidies, it is essential that the funds be allocated to (1) prospective students who otherwise would not have enrolled in the training program (marginal entrants) or (2) needy students who otherwise would not have completed their training (dropouts). Since it was very difficult to identify exactly who these individuals were, the NTA program had very little effect on either group and, therefore, very little impact on increasing the number of nurse graduates.

What the NTA program tried to do instead was to provide a financial reward to all recipients for a specific career relative to other careers. However, Professor Yett finds that neither the loan program nor the scholarship program was a major influence in raising the rate of return to nursing relative to other occupations.

Through further analysis, Professor Yett finds that two interrelated factors actually caused the sharp growth in the supply of active nurses despite the lack of a large increase in new graduates: (1) increases in the labor force participation rates of nurses, a supply response, and (2) large increases in nurse salaries caused by sharply increased demand for nurses due to the passage of Medicare and Medicaid.

In closing, Professor Yett cautions that, because of recent expansion and liberalization of the NTA program, its impact might become quite strong and be longlasting. He emphasizes that future policy decisions concerning the market for nurses must consider both the supply and demand side or the declining shortage of nurses might become a surplus.

Additional suggestions were made by some of the speakers concerning supply-side policies. Professor Schwartz offers two proposals to help correct the serious geographic and specialty maldistribution of physicians. One is the establishment of a national service for all young people which would require, for young graduating physicians, one to two years of service in some area of the United States with a shortage of physicians. The other is the establishment of a joint governmental-professional program which would establish criteria for reducing (increasing) the number of residencies for those specialties that have a surplus (shortage). Professors Feldstein and Kessel suggest methods to increase the supply and quality of health manpower—to increase supply, reduction of the training time required to qualify for a health profession, to increase quality, requirement of examinations at periodic intervals by health professionals for recertification. Professor Feldstein also calls for a reexamination of various state practice acts with an eye toward undoing barriers to entry. Professor Kessel also would like to see the opening up of state licensure examinations and/or national boards to all applicants regardless of how or where they received their training.

In closing, I would like to echo Professors Klarman and Schwartz by making two observations concerning the relationship between medical care delivery, the cost of medical care, and health. The first point is that the medical care delivery system, indeed medical care itself, is only one variable in a complex set which influences the health of an individual as well as a population. In many ways, environmental factors and individual life styles are much more important in determining health status than the medical care delivery system. Therefore, policies designed to alter medical care delivery may only have a modest effect on the actual health of the population. The other point is that the rising cost of medical care is in many ways linked to technological advances in medicine. For example, before insulin was discovered, the cost of treating diabetes was very low—the person simply died! With present day medicine, diabetes is fairly expensive to treat, but the patient is able to live. Clearly, then, we cannot focus our attention only on the costs of medical care but must also consider the major benefits that are received.

Acknowledgments

A novice at this sort of thing, I am very grateful to many people who helped me with the running of this seminar series and in the publication of this volume. Recognition is due to the members of the Department of

Economics at Western Michigan University for their acceptance of, and their general interest in, the series. Special thanks go to Dean Cornelius Loew, Associate Dean Tilman Cothran, and Professor Robert Bowers, Head of the Department of Economics, for their willingness to arrange the neccessary financial support. Thanks are also due to the members of the Lecture Series Committee during the 1973-74 academic year, Professors Werner Sichel and Wayland Gardner. The cooperation of the lecturers in the preparation of this publication is gratefully acknowledged, as is the interested participation of the students and the public who attended the lectures. Deep appreciation is expressed to Mrs. Em Hollingshead, Mrs. Cress Strand, and the Misses Pam Boerigter, Linda Kiser and Anita Shafer for their time, effort, and smiling faces while typing, retyping, and doing so many other necessary jobs associated with the preparation of the manuscript. Deep appreciation is also expressed for the expert editorial assistance provided by Mrs. Henrietta Slote of the Division of Research at the Graduate School of Business Administration, The University of Michigan. And last, but foremost, I wish to express sincere thanks especially to my wife, Betty, for her patience, understanding, and good cheer during all of the time that I was away from home.

Joseph C. Morreale

Western Michigan University
July, 1974

ABOUT THE SPEAKERS

PAUL FELDSTEIN *is a Professor in the Program in Hospital Administration in the School of Public Health at the University of Michigan and also Professor of Economics at the University. Under the auspices of a grant from the U.S. Public Health Services he directs a project to develop an econometric model of the medical care sector. He is also project director of a grant from the Robert W. Johnson Foundation to conduct studies of health manpower policies. Before joining the University of Michigan faculty in 1964, Dr. Feldstein directed the Division of Research of the American Hospital Association.*

Dr. Feldstein has held many advisory positions. He has served as consultant to the World Health Organization, Geneva (1972-73), and to the U.S. Bureau of the Budget and the Social Security Administration (1967-68). At present he is a consultant to the Commissioner for Social and Rehabilitative Services of Medicaid, to the Deputy Assistant Secretary for Health, HEW, and to the International Dental Study of the World Health Organization's National Institutes of Health, as well as to several other private and governmental organizations. He serves on the editorial board of Inquiry, *a publication of the Blue Cross Association, and is a fellow of the Institute for European Health Services Research (Louvain, Belgium).*

Dr. Feldstein has been a fellow of the W. K. Kellogg Foundation, and in 1969 he received the Edgar C. Hayhow Award from the American College of Hospital Administrators. A graduate of the College of the City of New York, he holds the M.B.A. and Ph.D. degrees from the University of Chicago. His numerous published articles have appeared in scholarly and professional reviews, in government journals, and in well-known textbooks.

HARRY SCHWARTZ, *a member of the editorial board of the* New York Times *since 1953, has served since 1969 on the faculty of the State University of New York at New Paltz, where he is designated*

Distinguished Professor. In 1973 he became Visiting Professor of Health Economics at Columbia University. A widely read author who has written on a diversity of subjects, Dr. Schwartz recently treated health economics in The Case for American Medicine *(McKay, 1972). He holds the B.A., M.A., and Ph.D. degrees from Columbia University.*

GERALD ROSENTHAL *is Director of the Bureau of Health Services Research, Washington, D.C. From 1973 through April 1974 he served as a public member and chairman of the Health Industry Wage and Salary Committee of the Cost of Living Council, Office of Wage Stabilization. Dr. Rosenthal has been Associate Professor on the faculty of Brandeis University, where he taught in the Department of Economics and the Florence Heller Graduate School of Social Welfare.*

Professor Rosenthal has actively served on committees and task forces to study health care industry matters for a wide range of governmental and private organizations, including the National Urban Coalition, the U.S. Public Health Service, the National Academy of Science, and the National Institute of Mental Health. From 1972 to 1973 he was President of the Massachusetts Public Health Association.

Dr. Rosenthal has presented papers at many professional conferences; his articles have also appeared in a wide range of periodicals; and he has contributed sections to several books, among them On Understanding Poverty: Perspectives from the Social Sciences, *edited by Daniel P. Moynihan (Basic Books, 1969). He is the author of* The Economics of Human Services *(Behavioral Press, 1974).*

DONALD E. YETT *is Director of the Human Resources Research Center at the University of Southern California, where he is also Professor of Economics and, in the University's Medical School, Professor of Community and Public Health. He has also served as Professor on the faculty of the University's Graduate School of Business Administration. A member of many professional associations, Dr. Yett is current chairman of the Health Economics Research Organization. He holds the B.A. and Ph.D. degrees from the University of Southern California.*

An active author, Professor Yett has presented papers at numerous national and international conferences, and his articles have been widely published in professional journals, in technical reports of governmental divisions, and in textbooks. His most recent book, An Economic Analysis of the Nurse Shortage, *is soon to be published by D. C. Heath and Company.*

He has been principal investigator or project director of many government grants to study different economic aspects of health care, among them policies to influence physicians' locational choice, the economic impact of alternative reimbursement programs, and manpower utilization in skilled nursing homes. Dr. Yett's present research interest focuses on an economic analysis of nursing services.

HERBERT E. KLARMAN *is Professor of Economics at the Graduate School of Public Administration, New York University.*

He is the author of two books, The Economics of Health *and* Hospital Care in New York City, *and the editor of* Empirical Studies in Health Economics. *He also has been a contributor to two textbooks for medical students. Author or coauthor of numerous articles on health planning, manpower, cost-benefit analysis, sources of increase in health care expenditures, and the HMO, Professor Klarman wrote many staff reports for the Hospital Council of Greater New York, of which he was Associate Director for twelve years.*

Professor Klarman teaches health planning, public expenditures analysis, and his specialty, health economics. He has taught at The Johns Hopkins University, Downstate Medical Center of the State University of New York, Columbia University, and Brooklyn College. He was educated at Columbia College and the University of Wisconsin.

A member of the Institute of Medicine of the National Academy of Science, Professor Klarman has served as a member of the Health Services Research Study Section, NIH, and on the U.S. National Committee on Vital and Health Statistics. He has been a consultant to the Bureau of the Budget, the Social Security Administration, and the National Center for Health Services Research and Development. Professor Klarman sits on the boards of editors of several journals.

REUBEN A. KESSEL *is Professor of Business Economics at the University of Chicago Graduate School of Business, where he joined the faculty in 1962, serving as Director of Research from 1969 to 1972. Professor*

Kessel has taught at the University of Missouri, the University of Southern California (Los Angeles), the University of Chicago Department Economics, and at the University of Washington (Seattle). He has also worked as an economist for industry and for private research organizations.

Dr. Kessel has written on a variety of economic subjects and many of his articles have been reprinted in distinguished textbooks and collected readings. His work as a researcher and professor has been recognized by awards from the Merrill Foundation for the Advancement of Financial Knowledge, the Volder Foundation, the Commission on Money and Credit, and the National Science Foundation.

THE PRESENT MEDICAL CARE SYSTEM IN THE UNITED STATES: AN ECONOMIC PROBLEM

PAUL FELDSTEIN

There are two basic issues in the debate over health care today. The first is equity in the distribution of medical care, i.e., how much medical care should be redistributed to those living in rural areas and to those of lower incomes. The second issue is one of efficiency. Are we getting our money's worth from the medical care system?

Some people might say that there is a third issue, namely, the effectiveness of medical care. Infant mortality rates in this country are higher than in some countries that spend less on their medical care system than we do. However, I believe that the concern with effectiveness is really a concern for efficiency: We are spending so much money, and are we any better off than other systems of delivery that spend less?

There are a number of legislative proposals that attempt to deal with equity and efficiency, either together or separately. Failure to separate the two issues can lead to confusion, since some people may disagree over the efficiency aspects of a proposal while others may differ on the amount to be spent to achieve greater equity. Furthermore, failure to separate these issues confuses the debate over how to achieve a given level of equity most efficiently. How much redistribution there should be is basically a value judgment. Some groups would prefer to provide minimum amounts of medical care to selected population groups together with minimum benefit coverage. Others would prefer unlimited access to medical care for everyone.

In my talk today therefore, I would like to separate the equity and efficiency issues and concentrate on the efficiency side, the delivery of medical care services. The first reason for emphasizing efficiency is that the cost of any equity objective and the ability to achieve it depend upon the efficiency and responsiveness of supply in meeting increased

1

demand—in this case, for medical care services. If demand for medical care increases as a result of government funding, then whether people will receive increased care will depend upon whether supply increases. If supply does not respond, then the increase in demand will merely lead to higher prices for medical care. If medical care prices rise rapidly, then the cost of medical care to people of middle and higher income levels will also increase, which will affect the willingness of middle and higher income groups to subsidize programs for lower income groups. It will also result in a demand by higher income groups for subsidies of their own medical care expenses.

The second reason for being concerned with the way medical care is delivered is that if supply is unresponsive then increased demand will lead to little increase in use and large price increases, and the cost of the program will become enormous. The cost to the government of redistribution programs is an important factor in considerations of how large such redistribution programs should be, how many people they should cover, and what benefits they should provide. The responsiveness of supply in medical care, therefore, will influence not only the program's cost and effectiveness but also its size. For example, many people will not favor a Kennedy-type national health insurance plan (which is very comprehensive in both its benefits and in the population covered), not because they disagree with the values inherent in such a plan, but because they believe its cost will be prohibitive.

Thus an examination of federal policies to increase the efficiency of the medical care sector becomes important because efficiency will determine whether or not a policy to increase demand will achieve its goal of increasing medical care to certain population groups and also what the cost and scope of proposed programs will be.

Before discussing the major policy options with respect to the organization and delivery of medical care, I would like to present some background on factors that have influenced the structure and organization of medical care.

Background

The hospital sector

Insurance for medical care started with coverage for just hospital care. Hospitalization was more unpredictable, the probable loss was greater, and the moral hazard involved was smaller than for other components of medical care. The type of hospital coverage first offered by the Blue Cross Association was a service benefit—i.e., full or nearly full coverage for the patient's hospital stay. The method of reimbursement under this arrangement was to the hospital and the amount was cost plus, that is, the hospital's cost plus a certain percentage for growth and development. Hospitals developed Blue Cross. And the service benefit to the patient and cost reimbursement to the hospital became a predominant form of insurance coverage for the United States. These Blue Cross concepts were later incorporated into most government financing programs for hospital care.

These insurance concepts of service-based cost reimbursement may be variously attributed to the value judgment that consumers are ignorant in the medical care marketplace (and their physician won't or can't choose for them). Alternatively, it may be said that it was really in the hospital's interest to have this form of reimbursement rather than one which would compel them to be more concerned with their prices relative to other institutions. For example, if patients received an indemnity benefit (in which case the patient is reimbursed directly by the insurance company and then he has to pay the hospital himself), then he (and his physician as his agent) would be more concerned with which hospital he enters and whether hospital care was the least costly way of treating his illness. Whether service-based cost reimbursement was a result of value judgments regarding the capability of the consumer or whether it was based on provider interest, it is now an essential feature of our medical care system.

This method of insurance reimbursement has led to the following problems: Any incentive to be concerned with costs which the patient or provider may have had was removed. Once the patient had hospital coverage, there was no need for him to shop around for a less costly hospital if he had to be hospitalized. The patient also had no incentive to be treated on an outpatient basis if Blue Cross paid his hospital care and he would have to pay the full price of outpatient care himself. Thus there was overuse of hospitals, which are the most costly component of medical care. Furthermore, since hospitals were reimbursed on the basis of their costs, they were able to expand, not in response to consumer demand, but because they could get reimbursed for whatever their costs were. In order to prevent the hospital system from expanding so rapidly, a control mechanism, other than consumer preference was needed. Thus, we had the development of hospital planning agencies. We will return to a discussion of planning later; at this point I just want to indicate why it has arisen and become an important policy strategy.

Because of cost-plus reimbursement to hospitals redistributive programs have become enormously costly. In 1966 Medicare and Medicaid were passed by the U.S. Congress. Medicare is a federal insurance program of hospital and physician care for the aged. Medicaid is a federal-state matching program for indigent populations, the level of indigency determined by each state. By 1971 annual public expenditures on Medicare and Medicaid had already climbed to over 13 billion dollars a year. This amount was much greater than anyone had imagined before the start of the programs. An important reason for the rapid rise in public expenditures under Medicare and Medicaid was the sharp increases in prices for hospital and physician services. In the period 1960-67, before the introduction of Medicare and Medicaid, hospital prices (daily service charges) rose 7.8 percent per year. After Medicare and Medicaid were started, hospital prices rose 16.6 percent the first year, 15.4 percent the second year, and between 12 and 13 percent for the subsequent years. A reason for the decline in the rates of increase was the economic stabilization program. Physician fees in the same period before Medicare and Medicaid rose at an annual rate of 3.5 percent per year. After the introduction of Medicare and Medicaid, physician fees rose between 6 percent and 7-1/2 percent per year. An important lesson from this experience is that any massive federal program that reimburses hospitals on the basis of cost and physicians on the basis of "reasonable and customary fees" is going to require an enormous amount of federal money, approximately $40 billion over a seven-year period, a large part of which was spent on higher prices rather than on more care.

We have thus far discussed the impact of past redistributive programs. Because of the lack of consumer incentives and the method of cost-based reimbursement, hospital costs and the cost to the government of redistribution programs have increased greatly. However, the nonprofit hospital sector is not the only one to blame. Other providers should also be assigned some responsibility for the higher cost of medical care and the increased cost of government redistribution programs.

While hospitals would prefer service benefits with cost reimbursement, physicians, on the other hand, would prefer indemnity-type insurance programs which would enable them to charge different patients more or less depending upon the family income. Thus, Blue Shield which was started by physicians, originally paid full coverage for physician care if the insured patient's income was under $7,500 a year. Once the patient's income was greater than $7,500, the physician could charge the patient more than just the Blue Shield payment for his service. Unlike the hospital, the physician would prefer to be reimbursed by the patient rather than directly by the insurance carrier. If the insurance carrier reimbursed the physician directly, then the physician could not charge more than a set payment and could not discriminate according to the patient's income. Thus, in order to get the cooperation of the American Medical Association for the passage of Medicare and Medicaid, the government allowed reimbursement to physicians on a "reasonable and customary fee" basis. Although there was some co-payment on the part of the patient, the entry of the government as a large payer on the basis of reasonable and customary fees enabled physicians to increase their fees greatly in the post-Medicare period. Since the number of physicians in the country cannot be changed very rapidly, physicians' incomes went up quite sharply.

Thus, although the hospital sector is primarily nonprofit and the physician sector can be considered as for profit, the price of care in each of these areas rose rapidly with the introduction of a large government redistribution program. As long as hospitals are reimbursed on the basis of their costs, no hospital will ever go out of business. The less efficient institutions not only survive but grow.

Redistributive programs become very costly because prices rise rapidly in the medical care market. These higher prices in turn cause cutbacks in government programs. For example, in many states, the Medicaid program, which is a state-federal matching program, was cut back, both in benefits provided and the population covered, because of the program's increased cost to the state.

The health professions

With regard to the various health professions—those of physicians, dentists, auxiliaries and technicians, and allied health personnel—there are numerous restrictions not only on who can enter each profession, but also on what tasks various people can perform. People are overtrained for what they do. The net result is that there are fewer health professionals, with higher incomes, than there would be if there were fewer restrictions. Under the guise of ensuring increased quality, health professionals have been instrumental in the passage of state laws (the medical and dental practice acts) which define who can practice and what tasks can be performed by what persons. Since a predominant reason for these restrictive practices is to increase the incomes of the health professionals themselves, the methods used to ensure high quality are all of the process type. That is, they emphasize the process of receiving high-quality training rather than the practice of high-quality care. Thus we find that persons wishing to practice medicine or dentistry must first be admitted to an approved school, then they must spend a minimum number of years in that institution (even though it has been shown that they can perform equally well when trained for shorter periods of time), and then they must pass an examination before they can become licensed. Once they are licensed, however, there is no periodic examination or monitoring of their practice to insure that high-quality care is retained or actually practiced. Such restrictions on who can enter the profession serve to decrease the supply of practitioners of that profession. Not everyone who wants to be or is qualified to be is admitted to the limited number of training spaces.

That these process measures for ensuring high quality merely serve to increase income by restricting supply becomes obvious when we observe how each profession treats foreign graduates. Since the rate of return in medicine or dentistry is so high in this country, it pays persons who cannot get admitted to the limited number of spaces here to go to schools outside of the country and then come back and practice here. This is also true for persons born and trained in other countries. Each profession tries to increase costs to the foreign-trained in order to decrease their rate of return in coming here. Citizenship requirements, which have nothing to do with quality, and additional educational requirements rather than just the use of examinations to measure proficiency are often imposed on this segment of potential practitioners.

Also passing under the guise of protecting consumers from low-quality care is the ban on advertising of price and quality of services by health professionals, their training, and refresher courses they may have taken. Prohibitions on such advertising only redound to the advantage of the profession since their effect is to allow the consumer less information on which to compare alternative providers.

The other health professionals are learning quickly from physicians and dentists. They also are lobbying for state laws that limit who can enter their professions and what tasks different professionals can do. There are currently more than 31 licensed health professions.

Another important sector of the health industry which is nonprofit and which has been the object of much federal and state financial support is that of the health profession educational institutions. It is here that we find important bottlenecks to increases in the supply of health manpower. There are several applicants for each space in medical and dental schools. Yet the health education industry grew at an incredibly slow pace before federal assistance finally tied the receipt of funds to increased enrollment. As long as schools were receiving unrestricted subsidies, why should they respond to market demands to produce more physicians and dentists? The reputation of medical and dental schools is not based on who produces more graduates but rather on who produces the highest quality physician or dentist. Again, because of the payment system to medical and dental schools, these schools are able to pursue their own goal which is to be prestigious institutions and they are immune from market pressures to produce more physicians and dentists.

This then is the market for medical care. It is predominantly non-profit—e.g., hospital and educational institutions—and the profit sector—physicians—is insulated from competitive pressures. These sectors have not been responsive to consumer demands nor have they been efficient in producing their product.

Lest we place our faith in other health care organizations to look out for our interests, we should consider the performance of intermediaries. The large payers of hospitals and physicians have been the insurance carriers, Blue Cross-Blue Shield, and the federal and state governments under Medicaid and Medicare. Past experience is again instructive as to the capability of these institutions to hold down costs. In the past, rather than monitor the adequacy of costs, these organizations have paid the bills that are rendered. In some instances, large nonprofit intermediaries have been criticized in congressional hearings for inadequacy in their own performance.

It appears, therefore, that the economic performance of the various sectors of the medical care industry has been pretty dismal. The nonprofit sectors have had a past history of being unresponsive to market demands and have experienced rapid increases in cost. The for-profit sectors have been able to construct legal barriers to prevent these professions from operating efficiently.

Restructuring of Supply: Policy Options

Thus unless there are changes in the delivery system it will not be possible to cover new population groups or to provide more medical care to those requiring it. Major structural changes in the organization and delivery of medical care become a prerequisite for the success of any new redistributive programs such as National Health Insurance.

In order to restructure the supply side we must first be explicit regarding the goals we would like to achieve. I believe that there are two objectives for policies on the supply side: The first is to make the supply side more responsive to consumer demands for medical care. The second is for the amount that is supplied to be produced as efficiently as possible. This would include using the right combination of hospital and outpatient care when possible.

What are our policy options in regard to restructuring the supply side of the medical care sector? One set of options is to impose a series of controls on hospitals, physicians, and the rest of the medical care sector. Along with such controls come proposals to pump more federal dollars into the health professions. The other broad set of policy options is to improve the market in which medical care is produced and provided. Both of these options are currently being pursued. However, it is unlikely that more than one strategy will prevail.

Control and regulation

I would like to discuss briefly each of these approaches. First, proposals for greater controls and regulation in the medical care markets, which involve both utilization review (PSROs) and planning.

Utilization review (PSROs). Partly as a result of the type of insurance coverage described earlier, which removes patient and physician incentives, and also because of inadequate monitoring of the quality of care actually practiced, federal legislation was passed setting up professional standard review organizations. This legislation, which the AMA very much opposes, requires peer review of medical utilization. The hope is that this will reduce both utilization and unnecessary medical care. However, other than utilization review procedures the general thrust of increased regulation is aimed at the supply side of the medical care sector.

Planning. In the past a number of hospital planning agencies have been established with federal funds. Their efforts to improve the allocation of hospital beds and services in an area have consisted of working with the hospitals concerned for voluntary compliance with their plans; they have had no power to enforce their decisions on the local hospitals, and such efforts to limit construction and duplication of facilities and services have been a failure. Since the support of the local hospitals was generally required for continuance of financial support to the planning agency from the government, vigorous action on the part of the local hospital planner could and did lead to his premature departure.

In an attempt to strengthen the planning agency, a number of states are passing certificate-of-need legislation, which requires prior approval from the appropriate hospital planning agency for expansion of beds in a hospital. Certificate-of-need legislation is generally favored by existing hospitals and, of course, by Blue Cross. Existing hospitals would favor such legislation, because limits on expansion essentially preclude new competitors from entering the area. Blue Cross would favor it because its main effect is to decrease or hold down the number of hospital beds and, therefore, hospital utilization. With such legislation in effect Blue Cross premiums would not rise as rapidly and it would thus be more competitive with commercial insurance companies.

Certificate-of-need legislation has several potential drawbacks. First, it does not deal with the problem of cost control; it is just a capital control program. In fact, one study measuring the impact that hospital planning agencies have had on hospital costs found that the increase in annual costs was as high in communities with planning agencies as in communities without such agencies. If hospitals are precluded from entering an area, then existing high-cost hospitals would be less concerned with their patients' having alternative institutions to go to. A second drawback of certificate-of-need legislation is that limiting the number of hospitals in an area may hamper the development of Health Maintenance Organizations (HMOs)—a form of prepaid medical care that requires the organization either to have its own hospital or to contract with an existing hospital so as to be able to provide hospital coverage. Thus the existing fee-for-service system in an area could effectively eliminate the competitive threat of HMOs by denying them the ability to construct their own hospitals or to contract with existing hospitals. A third drawback is that existing institutions have not always served the poor or the minority groups in the areas in which they are located. Neighborhood health centers sponsored by federal funds have been developed to serve those groups. Restricting the development of new institutions by certificate of need is likely to decrease accessibility to medical care to certain population groups, which would be contrary to the objective of much of our redistributive policy.

Underlying these hypothesized effects is a basic assumption that the existing institutions will effectively control the local planning agency so that it will operate in their behalf. Past experience with such agencies lends support to this hypothesis. In this regard it is instructive to examine the behavior of other regulatory agencies in our society—federal agencies, such as the ICC and the CAB, and agencies within the medical field itself, such as medical and dental examining boards. It is difficult to find many instances when these agencies have acted contrary to the interest of the group they are intended to regulate. It is my belief that hospital planning agencies strengthened with certificate-of-need legislation will be no different.

It is also popular today to suggest that hospitals be treated as public utilities, although hospitals do not have any of the economic characteristics of public utilities, namely that it is efficient to have only one firm serving an area. The possible savings, if any, of having one large hospital serving the community would be more than offset by the decrease in its accessibility. Another explanation for the hospitals' desire for public-utility status is that it will ensure the survival of existing hospitals. No public utility commission forces the utility it controls out of business. Instead, it insures that the utility receives a fair "rate of return."

Rate regulation. The third set of controls is rate regulation. The first two forms of regulation, utilization review and certificate of need, serve to reduce utilization. Therefore, another form of regulation is required to hold down rising costs and prices. Under the Economic Stabilization Program prices are slowly being decontrolled. However, the health sector controls are likely to remain. The cost and price controls are specified at a federal level, but states are encouraged to set up their own regulatory agencies. The federal controls on hospitals have had an effect. As described earlier the annual increase in hospital prices before the introduction of Medicare and Medicaid was approximately 6 percent per year. After Medicare and Medicaid hospital prices increased at an annual rate of 16 percent per year. Thereafter it increased between 12 percent and 13 percent per year until the economic stabilization program became effective and reduced annual price increases to only 6.6 percent per year—a 50 percent reduction. (When the increase in hospital costs are examined, the effect of the control program was to decrease the rise in hospital costs by 20 percent and 25 percent from 14 percent to 9 percent per year.)

Price and cost controls work. But they are no panacea to the problem of rising hospital costs and adequate health care. If the objective is to reduce the rise in hospital costs, then such controls can be effective. But there is a risk that the controls will be arbitrarily or politically determined. Hospitals may be forced to make reductions in the scope and quality of their services and to narrow the range of population groups they serve. The net effect might be to lower costs for hospital care but to produce a program which was costly in other respects.

Hospitals have, of course, been against the continuance of such cost controls. As an alternative they have favored prospective reimbursement, a form of voluntary budget review between each hospital and Blue Cross. Although slow to start, a number of experiments in this area have begun. To date there is no evidence that such a review process results in lower annual cost increases. Furthermore, the experience of other countries, such as Sweden and England, with similar budget review mechanisms, shows that hospital costs have increased at least as rapidly as in this country.

Thus, voluntary efforts to hold down annual cost increases have not been, nor are they likely to be, successful. The above types of control and regulation do not address any of the restrictions on the supply of health personnel. Minimum educational requirements, licensing boards controlled by the professionals themselves, and restrictions on tasks are not considered, nor are they likely to be, in a system that becomes more regulated. If there is a shortage of health professionals then the approach under such a system is to fund large programs to increase the supply of these professionals. No changes are made in the structure of the system that produces them or in the conditions under which they practice. Large funding programs to decrease shortages of health manpower essentially mask the large inefficiencies that exist in the market for producing such personnel.

Improvement of the market

Well, what can be done to improve the organization and delivery of medical care? An alternative to increasing controls and regulation is to improve the various markets for medical care. Specifically, the consumer should be permitted access to information on provider performance, quality, and prices. The consumer cannot but benefit from such additional information. Consumers are ignorant when it comes to their treatment needs and they have to rely on physicians. However, this is insufficient reason for prohibiting suppliers from providing information to them. As long as some consumers can use this information to make choices—and there are some very large and knowledgable consumers such as unions—then it will benefit all other consumers as well. For example, one study of prices paid for prescription eyeglasses found that in states where advertising was permitted the average price paid was lower and the range of prices paid was smaller than in those states where advertising was prohibited. Prohibition of advertising in medical care may be based on the belief that all consumers are incapable of using information. This assessment of consumers is a value judgment which has not, in my opinion, been empirically verified in the health field. Even in the complex area of insurance benefits, we find that utilization patterns follow insurance benefits, suggesting that consumers seek out information and use it to their advantage. The only other reason for not permitting advertising in medical care is that the providers are against it. It is considered "unethical" behavior. It is clear why providers would be against permitting advertising, but it is not obvious why consumers should be willing to go along with what is in the providers' interest but not in their own.

The second major change I would like to see in the medical sector is a re-examination of the various practice acts in each state. Current practice acts for the health professions define who can and cannot practice and also what tasks are permitted by other health professionals. These practice acts are always administered by the profession that is regulated. A large degree of public representation should be consolidated with professional representation in the administration of the various acts. This change will, I hope, eliminate many of the restrictions placed on different professions.

Furthermore, the emphasis on the process requirements for maintaining high quality should be changed. Minimum educational requirements should not be required; instead the emphasis should be placed on examinations and on monitoring the quality of care practiced. Quality control should be a continual process and not based on a one-time licensure examination.

A third change along the same lines should be a reduction in the training times to qualify for a health profession. Many skilled health professionals are overtrained for the tasks they actually perform, and there is no upward mobility in the health professions. One important reason why there are shortages of health personnel in certain areas is that it does not pay a person with so many years of training to practice in less desirable areas when he could earn much more elsewhere.

A case in point is the claim that there is a shortage of family practitioners. The proposed policy for easing this shortage is to establish new training programs in family practice which will consist of a three-year residency after graduation from medical school. However, the reasons most often given for the decline of family practitioners is that family practice is boring and it doesn't pay as well as other medical specialities. It is boring because the type of patients seen are routine and any interesting cases are referred to specialists. If the same amount of training were required for family practice as for other specialties, a family practitioner could enter one of the other specialties and have a much higher income. The proposed approach, therefore, should be not to increase the residency training period for family practitioners but instead to reduce it. Because of the limited nature of the practice the physician can be trained in a shorter period of time. He does not have to learn all of the science areas that he will never have occasion to use, that he will probably forget, and for which he will, in any case, refer his patient to a specialist. Secondly, decreasing the training time for family practitioners will increase their rate of return. A family physician can start practicing sooner than one who goes on for speciality training, which will make family practice more remunerative.

Nor does every doctor need to be trained to do the same thing. Doctors could be given limited licenses. Such an approach would require a change in medical school education, because the objective of medical school educators now, rather than being to train large numbers of physicians, is to train a few physicians who have national and international reputations.

The final major change I would like to see in the medical care market is one which is beginning to occur and which may have more likelihood of success than the changes I suggested previously—that is, the development of HMOs. Many state laws passed at the instigation of the AMA have thus far retarded the development of HMOs in this country, and such forms of practice were further hampered by local AMA efforts to deny hospital staff privileges to physicians wishing to participate in this form of practice. In the past few weeks, however, the U. S. Congress passed legislation on HMOs. In addition to providing subsidies to such organizations the federal legislation preempts state laws that inhibit their development. Prepaid medical care, which both political parties support, although they still differ on the structure of HMOs and on minimum benefit packages, can be expected to become an important method of delivery of medical care in the next decade.

The hoped-for advantage of HMOs is that there will be greater incentive to be efficient in the delivery of medical care than in the current fee-for-service system. Since the organization receives a specified premium per family and not cost reimbursement, the organization has an incentive to produce its services as efficiently as possible. It also has the incentive not to use more costly forms of institutional care, such as hospitals, if less costly care will suffice. Further, faced with a budgetary constraint of a fixed premium per year, the HMO would not have any reason to provide unnecessary services nor duplicate facilities and services that currently exist in the community. If responsibility for quality can be shifted from licensing agencies within each health profession to the institution itself, then there can be greater use of less-skilled persons in the delivery of care. The HMOs in an area should serve as a competitor to the existing fee-for-service system. Such competition should not only provide the consumer with more choice than has previously existed, but should also hopefully result in cost and quality competition in the medical care market.

Because of the time constraint to my talk, I have touched briefly upon many complex areas. In conclusion, therefore, I would like to emphasize that differences in policy options as to how our medical care system is to be restructured are, in part, a result of value judgments such as how much medical care should be redistributed and under what conditions, and also a result of how the consumer is viewed: Is he capable of choosing rationally given more information? Differences in policy strategies are also due to differences over how to achieve greater efficiency in the delivery of medical care services. It is clear that major redistributive programs cannot be undertaken until the supply side of the medical care market is made more responsive. Otherwise new financing programs will merely increase prices to everyone (especially those not included in the financing program) as well as an increase the cost of the program to the government.

The major policy alternatives for restructuring the organization and delivery of medical care are (1) to institute more controls and regulations in the payment and delivery of medical care services or, conversely, (2) to reduce the restrictions on entry into the health professions and on tasks persons can perform and to offer alternative forms of delivery, such as HMOs, among which consumers can choose. Both systems cannot operate together. Controls and regulations in my opinion cannot respond to consumer preferences. They cannot achieve efficiency in the delivery of care. Permitting the corporate practice of medicine through HMOs will, I hope, provide an opportunity to organize the industry more efficiently by introducing cost incentives among providers. In sponsoring the development of HMOs we should provide them with greater responsibility for the quality of medical care (and we should monitor the care they provide) by letting them determine the tasks persons can perform and the training necessary to learn those tasks rather than letting each health profession determine its own education and licensing requirements.

THE CASE FOR AMERICAN MEDICINE

HARRY SCHWARTZ

It is an interesting commentary on our times that it is necessary for somebody to write a book, as I have done, and give a lecture, as I intend to do this evening, with a title even remotely approximating "The Case For American Medicine." I am a little uncomfortable about the title because it suggests that in some sense I think there is something good about being sick. I do not. I want to emphasize that at the very beginning; above all else it is better to be healthy. Unfortunately we can not control the state of our health all of the time. All of us will be sick and all of us, of course, will die.

Now, what also interests me is that there are very few people, at least among the fairly articulate, who have much good to say about American medicine today. We live in a period when, in general, it is fashionable to be extremely critical of American institutions. A combination of the Viet Nam war and Watergate has produced a great deal of disillusionment, disenchantment, and cynicism about all aspects of American society. American medicine, in particular, has been a special victim of this disenchantment for several years. When one goes to the library and searches through the shelves of books on American medicine, what one normally finds is that all of the books, whatever their titles, come down to the case against it. As a matter of fact until I wrote my book, there was almost no book that had a kind word to say for American medicine, which is perhaps a commentary in itself. Even before the current disenchantment, let's say five years ago, we had a CBS television show "Don't Get Sick in America," which was an attack on American medicine. I always wondered where was a good place to get cancer, or where was it wise to get multiple sclerosis or schizophrenia? I do not know. The idea, "don't get sick in America," with its implication that some other place is paradise, where, perhaps, you can get cancer happily, makes no sense to me at all.

15

Now why is there so much criticism of American medicine by many who argue that revolutionary changes must be made in the American medical system? Senator Kennedy has had a very sweeping national health insurance bill before Congress for several years, one which in the opinion of many observers—although he himself denies it—would go far toward socializing the American system. There are other bills before Congress of somewhat lesser scope. At any rate, the feeling that very radical change is necessary is rather widespread in some influential circles. One would be foolish to ignore it.

Common Criticisms of American Health Care

In order to understand this phenomenon one has to know the chief arguments made against American medicine, which can be summarized very briefly. First, it has been charged that American medical care is poor and that the health of the American people is deficient. The critics point to statistics comparing the United States to many other nations of the world, data that show that we are approximately twentieth in the world in infant mortality and perhaps twenty-fifth in length of life. The critics appear to argue that the medical system here just does not work and the American people are very sick people. Then, second, there is the related argument that this country has a terrible doctor shortage. In reading some of the critics you get the impression that nobody ever gets to see a doctor. Yet, government statistics show that in 1973 there were something like one billion patient-doctor contacts outside of hospitals in the United States. That is, one billion times a year in this country doctors and patients got together in one way or another, which comes to about five times per person on the average. And yet a lot of the material presented by the critics sounds as though you never can get a doctor. A hallowed figure that is often presented is the contention that we have a shortage of 50,000 doctors. This number was first enunciated about 1956; since that year the number of doctors in the United States has increased by more than 100,000. Nevertheless, I keep on reading about a 50,000-doctor shortage.

A third argument presented by the critics is that there is a maldistribution of medical services throughout the country. Many rural areas and many urban ghetto areas have few or no physicians, we are told, and lack necessary medical facilities, a situation that is denounced in very eloquent and very vivid language. Finally, the critics complain that medical care here is terribly expensive. A typical recent cartoon in the *New Yorker* showed a patient sitting in a hospital corridor in front of a hospital room. He had a hat in one hand and a sign in the other which said, "$135 a day. Please help." The expense argument is frequently reinforced by horror stories of one sort or another about patients made bankrupt by large medical bills. What clearly emerges from these critiques, which are usually expressed much more dramatically and in a much more emotional form than I have used, is that the whole edifice is rotten, we must get rid of it, and we have to create a shining new medical utopia.

The shining new medical utopia that is normally urged rests on two basic assumptions. One, health care is a right. This is a very emotional slogan, which apparently implies that everyone should get àll the health care he wishes free of charge, anytime he wants it, and wherever he wants it. And second, the entire fee-for-service system should be wiped out and instead physicians should become directly, or indirectly, government employees and required to practice in a certain mode. The currently fashionable mode is called the Health Maintenance Organization, which is essentially the well-known system of prepaid group practice and its variants. If we just have the wit, we are told, we can escape the clutches of the AMA, and we can get into this beautiful, magical medical utopia. I hope the critics don't think I am being unfair, but I have tried to start by enunciating what I think are the main criticisms of the medical systems.

Refutations

Let me begin again by saying that no reasonable person can deny there are deficiencies in American medicine. I would go even further and say that there are deficiencies in all American institutions. I suspect there might even be deficiencies in Western Michigan University. No person can work in an institution without seeing its problems. I take for granted that there are inadequacies and that things can be improved in American medicine as in all other American institutions. Moreover, I also take for granted that in a nation of 210 million people where you have in one year a billion doctor-patient contacts outside of hospitals, one can find horror stories which depict unhappy, unpleasant, and even tragic incidents in the delivery of medical care. Having granted all that, I think there is another side of the story, and what bothers me is that this other side of the story is so rarely presented. We seem to be seized with such a mood of negativism about America and about its institutions and its society that we fail to realize there are many positive aspects. And I would add that there is a great deal that is positive about the American medical system.

The first question that comes to mind is, if things are really so dreadful here, why do you people look so healthy? I think that much of the discussion of United States medical care is an example of misrepresentation. I do not mean to suggest that it is intended, but nevertheless, it has resulted. It is misrepresentation based upon emphasizing the unrepresentative. That is, the simple truth is that the great majority of Americans are healthy. Moreover, insofar as modern science knows how to, it has eradicated much disease. After all, remember that my generation recalls that, when our kids were small, every year from April to October we lived in absolutely constant fear, because every year this country had a polio epidemic. Now, I discover that the present generation of college students, for the most part, has never heard of polio. Polio is now a historical disease. If you look at the data, you find that in a typical recent year this country of 210 million people has had perhaps a half dozen or a dozen polio cases. To somebody in my generation, this is an absolute miracle. So I would argue that there has been a tremendous amount of progress.

This progress is also evident in the present concern about the population problem. If the health of the United States were so dreadful, if everybody were so sick and everybody were dying prematurely, would we need to discuss the importance of zero population growth? Why do we have to legalize abortion? Why do we have to popularize the use of contraceptives? The answer is very simple: the advances in sanitation, and in environment, and in nutrition, etc., plus medical advances, have eradicated many of the killers which kept the old equilibrium. It is precisely because the probability of a newborn baby's living to adulthood is now so high that we have to find artificial means of controlling population. If the medical system and the health of the United States were as bad as it's supposed to be, there would be no need for a ZPG movement. ZPG, without people's realizing it, is a testimonial to how healthy people really are.

I would also argue that the medical data show clearly the relative good health of the United States population, if you look at this data with sophisticated eyes. When people tell you how bad American health is, you must ask them, "With whom are you comparing us?" Two favorite countries to which the United States is compared are Iceland and Sweden. But the difficulty with such comparisons is that Iceland has only 200,000 people and Sweden only 8 million. Now, what sense does it make to compare the United States with 210 million people to the 200,000 people in Iceland, or to the 8 million people in Sweden? The one country with which the United States is probably really comparable in terms of being a large country, in terms of being a country with a heterogeneous population, an industrialized country in which extensive medical resources are known and available, is the Soviet Union. And the Soviet Union, in addition, has a socialized medical system.

In a certain sense, medical care is "free" in the Soviet Union. Although, of course, there is nothing free in the world, and all the word "free" means is that in the Soviet Union the medical system is paid for through taxes. Yet when you compare the U.S. figures, whether on infant mortality, or length of life, etc., with the Soviet figures, you discover something very interesting: the U.S. figures are better. Infant mortality in the United States is lower than in the Soviet Union, and the U.S. life expectancy is longer. So, many of the arguments telling us about how dreadful health is in the United States are really arguments based upon statistical naïveté. They are also based on statistical trickery, and they carefully ignore the vast advances the United States has made in recent years in lowering infant mortality and increasing the length of life.

Another point to be made about the United States is that it is quite clear that if you are going to be sick, particularly if you get a serious illness, no nation matches the United States in terms of the availability of first-class medical care. It is simple truth that in terms of the number and competence of the people available to do the job, or the availability of the expensive equipment needed, the United States is in a class by itself. Let me give just a few examples which are indicative of the total situation. Take the case of Louis Russell, Jr. Louis Russell, Jr. is a black vocational high school instructor who is about 47 years of age now and lives in Indianapolis, Indiana. Five and one-half years ago, Louis Russell, Jr. was dying of a serious heart ailment. He was sent by his doctor in Indianapolis to the Medical College in Richmond, Virginia, in order to undergo a heart transplant. That was 5½ years ago, and Louis Russell, Jr. is still alive and living a full life. I spoke to him last August on the fifth anniversary of his heart transplant, and he told me that in the average week he makes three or four speeches. He sounded like a very vigorous, very healthy guy over the phone, and his pictures make him look very good. Now, it seems to me that when you have a man who has lived with a transplanted heart and lived well, not an invalid, for 5½ years you are describing some kind of a miracle. Louis Russell, Jr. is by far the longest-lived heart transplant patient in the world.

But an additional point emerges from this example. Louis Russell, Jr., did not go to the top heart transplant team in the world. That honor belongs to the team of Dr. Norman Shumway at Stanford University. Most of the people who are alive today with transplanted hearts which are beating and working are Norman Shumway's patients. So it is quite clear that Louis Russell, Jr., is a victory for the people at the Medical College of Virginia in the era of heart transplants on a worldwide scale, and the victory was achieved by a United States team not even comparable to the team at Stanford University. And the United States does not just lead in heart transplants, it is also the leader in kidney transplants. The great majority of the more than 10,000 kidney transplants in the world have been done right here in the United States. The best results by far, have been obtained in the United States. So if you have a bad kidney your chances of getting good care and surviving are much better in the United States than any place else. By and large, this is true of most serious illnesses which occur in human beings.

The United States, I repeat, has many more highly trained physicians, nurses, and technicians, and more complex equipment and hospitals than any other nation. We are in a better position to give highly specialized, highly skilled care than any other country. The Soviet Union recognized that fact recently. Soviet authorities turned to this country to meet the medical needs of a very highly placed Soviet scientist, Mikkail Keldysh, who was very ill. Academician Keldysh is the president of the Soviet Academy of Sciences and he is also in charge of the Soviet space program. Obviously a very important man in the Soviet Union, Academician Keldysh was dying of a heart ailment a year ago. The Soviet government, desperate to save Professor Keldysh's life, sent for Dr. Michael DeBakey of Houston, Texas. Dr. DeBakey flew twice from Houston to Moscow and performed two major operations on Dr. Keldysh, and Dr. Keldysh is presently doing very well. DeBakey's feat was so enormous that *Pravda* publicly thanked him for what he had done for the president of the Soviet Academy of Sciences. Some of you may also remember information that became known a few years ago when Nikita Khrushchev's memoirs were being published by *Life* magazine. This was the news that when a member of Khrushchev's family was very sick, the Soviet leader sent for a doctor from Johns Hopkins University in Baltimore, Maryland. So, these examples reveal that among connoisseurs of medical care, it is well known that by far the finest care in the world is available in the United States. I repeat, there is no place where it is good to get sick. Being healthy is better, but if you do get sick there is no better care available anywhere than there is here in the United States. This fact should make one very cautious about radical change in the medical care system. A society which produces the best quality medical care for serious illnesses has much in its favor, and one ought to be careful about meddling with this very complex system.

Well, what about the charge that there is a terrible doctor shortage? I find there is a very widespread notion that some kind of monopoly controls the supply of doctors. Well, this whole argument is absolutely nonsense. Within less than the past decade the number of places for medical students in American medical schools has risen by about 50 percent. Every year for the past decade, the number of people graduating from medical school has set a new high record. Moreover, large numbers of foreign-trained physicians enter this country each year, and many settle here permanently. In general, the total number of physicians in this country has, in recent years, grown by about three times the rate of the population's growth. Very roughly speaking, the number of physicians has been increasing by about 3 percent a year, while the population has been increasing by only about 1 percent a year. Moreover, in the last couple of years we have had a very drastic drop in the birth rate with, of course, an accompanying drop in the rate of population growth. Therefore, we are seeing the phenomenon of the population's growth slowing down perceptibly, while the growth in the number of physicians continues to accelerate. This trend has prompted the Assistant Secretary of Health, Education, and Welfare, Dr. Charles Edwards, speaking last November before the convention of medical colleges in Washington, to declare that in his view we are on the verge of a surplus of physicians. This statement really surprised me because I thought that the words "doctor shortage" had become absolutely obligatory in the United States. How often, after all, does reality intrude into the comments of a high government official?

Now, what I have been arguing essentially is that there is a great deal of good quality medical care in this country. A great deal of medical care is given, much is given quite expertly, and much is given quite sympathetically. The United States is not a medical wasteland. I also contend that much of the contrary argument totally misrepresents the United States medical care system.

Health maintenance organizations

Let us turn now to one proposed remedy for the alleged deficiencies of the fee-for-service, free enterprise medical system, namely the Health Maintenance Organization (HMO). It is argued that the cost of the fee in the fee-for-service system inhibits or precludes people from going to the doctor in time. Allegedly, sick people only go to the doctor when their illness is in an advanced stage, and then the medical costs are high. It is claimed that HMOs would remedy this situation. The HMO prepaid group practice is a system which at least is exemplified by Kaiser-Permanente. A fixed sum, say $500, is paid for each person per year. Then this person can go to the doctor whenever he wishes and receive all his medical care "free of charge" beyond the basic charge. So it appears that since the out-of-pocket is zero, the above inequity is remedial.

In answer to the critics, I would like to refer to some recent statements by the founder of the Kaiser-Permanente scheme, in a sense the founder of the HMOs, Dr. Sydney Garfield. I refer you to one of the most readily available of his writings, an article in the *Scientific American* for April 1970. I paraphrase his ideas about fee for service. He claims that when he and his associates started Kaiser-Permanente they thought that the fee for service was the obstacle to medical care. They substituted the capitation

system, the prepaid system, so that the cost of the fee would not be a
barrier to medical care. Dr. Garfield now says that after thirty years of
experience with this system they have discovered that the absence of a fee
is as much of a barrier as the fee was. And why? Because in the real world
we always live between Scylla and Charybdis. The critics choose to
emphasize Scylla: Some Americans may not go to a doctor when they
ought to because of the need to pay a fee. But that is only one rock, only
one side of the picture. But what is forgotten is the rock on the other side.
When people are not charged an out-of-pocket fee, you get flooded by
what Dr. Garfield calls the "worried well." I once said that he means the
hypochondriacs, but he responded that the worried well were a much
bigger group than hypochondriacs. What Dr. Garfield says is that when
you do not have a fee for service, the "worried well" flood the system, they
"usurp" the resources needed to treat the genuinely ill, and the genuinely
ill suffer.

I do not want to give you the impression that the fee-for-service system
is perfect. I am sure that the fee for service sometimes keeps people from
needed access. Although, of course, in our society with Medicaid and
Medicare and numerous hospital clinics, I think in a large city or city area
you have to be pretty uninformed not to figure out how to see a doctor
without paying for it. Certainly, in New York City that is true. When you
remove the fee from service, what you do is you open the doctor's door to
all of the large number of "worried well" people. A very important point
to bear in mind is that most of the people that a general practitioner sees
daily have nothing organically wrong with them. A very large portion of
those people who go to physicians in this country go because they are lone-
ly, because they just want to talk to a doctor. A tremendous amount of
money in this country is wasted every year on elaborate tests and x-rays
for people who have nothing organically wrong with them.

So the fee for service is at least a motive for economy. When you take it
away, you have an incentive to waste. How you balance the two is a difficult question, but one ought to be aware that there are both problems.
Therefore, I do not see the HMO, prepaid system as the cure-all it is made
out to be.

Suggested Solutions to the Real Weaknesses
of the Health Care System

Now having said that, I want to point out that, of course, there are real
weaknesses in the United States medical care system. Not all of the com-
plaint is imaginary by any means. As I said before, I think that in terms of

a total number of doctors we have more than enough and we do not have a shortage. What we do have is a serious maldistribution of doctors. In a city like San Francisco, you may well have 50 percent more doctors than are needed for that area. On the other hand in many rural areas and in some ghetto areas you have an inadequate number of doctors or no physicians at all. We certainly do have a geographic maldistribution, and we also have a specialty maldistribution. We need more primary care physicians, which includes general practitioners, family physicians, internists, and pediatricians. We almost certainly have too many surgeons. Clearly, something needs to be done about these maldistributions.

The problem in rural areas can be solved by a national service for all young people, perhaps along the lines that they have in Israel. Such a program would require every young person graduating from college or of a certain age to give one or two years of his or her life to some socially useful project. In the case of young graduating physicians, after their internship year, they would be required to serve in areas which require a physician, such as rural areas. This particular geographic maldistribution cannot be corrected by the free market, fee-for-service system. The problem is that physicians do not like rural areas; the areas lack intellectual and professional stimulation and their educational systems are poor. Now it may be that the pollution in the big cities is getting so bad that tastes may change and many people, including doctors, will be rushing out to the rural areas. But up to this point, this has not been true.

Turning to the ghetto areas, I think that the main cause for the lack of physicians here is simple physical security. From a free market fee-for-service point of view, some of the most profitable practices in the country are in ghetto areas. In Washington, D.C., a black obstetrician in a black ghetto area collected $250,000 last year just from Medicaid, and this amounted to less than half his practice. The *Washington Post* looked into his practice and found that he was doing a high quality job. He was seeing a large number of patients; he had very modern equipment; he had five highly trained assistants. The *Post*'s original reaction was that this doctor must be some kind of a crook, but when they investigated his practice, they came away writing two very admiring articles about this physician. This example shows that the fee-for-service system has rewards under Medicaid that would attract many people into the ghetto areas. Yet, a lot of people are afraid, many with a good deal of cause, that they may be killed. And doctors have been killed in ghetto areas. So I think the problem remains one of security.

What is the solution to distribution of specialty physicians? There is a major problem attached to the correction of maldistribution. The medical profession is very slow, perhaps too show, to alter the number of residencies for each specialty. There have been a lot of legal opinions to the effect that if the medical profession itself tried to do something about the supply of residencies it would be in violation of the anti-trust laws. In other words, let us say that the American College of Surgeons announces that it is going to cut the number of surgical residencies because there are too many surgeons. They might very well be prosecuted under the anti-trust laws. Actually, I think, if there were some kind of joint governmental-professional program which received exemption from the anti-trust laws, the problem could easily be solved. The government would have to see that the public interest was protected. This joint public-private enterprise program could establish criteria for reducing the number of residencies in those specialities where there is a surplus and increasing the number of residencies in those specialities where there is a shortage. The exact criteria would have to be worked out but, in principle at least, such a program could be undertaken.

Now what about the problem of the high cost of medical care? Well, the average American family tends to be a pretty healthy family which has no trouble meeting its medical bills. The data are all there and quite evident. Now the problem of cost comes up. When you contract a serious illness you have to spend a long while in the hospital. Fortunately, most Americans have hospital insurance. About 90 percent of the population has some form of hospitalization insurance. Moreover, many Americans are also covered by government programs like Medicare and Medicaid. So, there is a tremendous amount of protection in insurance in the United States and, in a sense, this is one of our problems. We have lost the incentive to economize on hospital care, which *is* expensive, not only here but in all countries.

For many people the cheapest kind of care is hospital care. I, for example, like millions of Americans, have a Blue Cross policy which provides for 120 days of hospital care a year. The minute I enter a hospital it does not cost me a penny for 120 days except if I want to make phone calls, or have a television set in my room, or want a newspaper. Otherwise, it does not cost me anything. One of our problems as a result is that certain kinds of care are too cheap. We do not treat them economically because they do not require immediate out-of-pocket payment; we demand them excessively. As a matter of fact, this excess demand—particularly stimulated by Medicare and Medicaid which were adopted less than a decade ago—has played a very important role in forcing up prices in medical care. And most of you probably know that from 1965 on, for about a half a decade, medical care prices were the most rapidly rising prices in the American marketplace.

But is this rapid inflation in the medical care market still continuing?

The critics would have you think so, but it is no longer true.[1] After August 1971, when President Nixon established the wage and price control program, the one area in which that program definitely worked was the area of medical costs. The index of medical prices in the consumer price index reported by the Bureau of Labor Statistics has been the most slowly rising major element in the entire cost-of-living index spectrum. This fact is particularly evident in the last year or two, when one compares the rise in food and fuel prices with the rise in medical prices. In effect then, an interesting change has occurred which has been given very little public attention: the inflation of medical care costs, caused by Medicare and Medicaid originally, has been abruptly halted.

As a matter of fact, the rise in hospital prices has been held back so much that a great many hospitals claim that they are near bankruptcy. And the American Hospital Association filed suit against the price control authorities on the ground that the controls were driving a large segment of the American hospital economy into bankruptcy. I do not know whether this allegation is true or not, but what is certainly true is that August 1971, represented a historic divide in the recent trend of medical care prices.

The problem of rising medical costs is clearly coming under control. But the problem of overwhelming medical bills still remains. To solve this problem, we need catastrophic medical insurance. For example, if you had the bad luck to get leukemia, in the past it was often not an economic catastrophe, because leukemia killed you very quickly. However, because of the progress of science and technology in medicine, if you get leukemia now, very frequently you can last for years and years. As a matter of fact, you can even have periods of long-standing remission in which you live more or less a normal life. But this increased ability to live carries with it enormous cost, because of the long period of care required. The same thing is true for many other diseases, such as many types of cancer or heart disease. These are catastrophic illnesses about which we know enough now to prolong life, often at very high costs, but unfortunately not enough to cure the disease. Clearly, when you get some of these terrible illnesses, there is no question that the medical expenses are very large and will rapidly surpass the total benefits that most health insurance policies will cover. Well, the answer to this problem is very clear: catastrophic medical insurance.

I find it very interesting that for more than a decade now Senator

---

[1]The reader should bear in mind that Professor Schwartz's remarks were made before the lifting of the wage and price control program in May 1974. At this writing it is evident that inflation will again become a major problem in the medical care market. This result might indicate that President Nixon's program only postponed the inevitable increases in medical care prices and really was not a success.—Ed.

Russell Long of Louisiana has been trying to push a plan for catastrophic insurance and has not been successful in getting it enacted. Both the right and the left are opposed to catastrophic insurance, and it is interesting to know their reasons. The left is opposed because the most frequent horror stories about the alleged sins of American medicine usually have to do with a case of catastrophic illness. One very clear example of such a story occurred when President Lyndon Johnson's brother Sam went into bankruptcy because some orthopedic problem forced him to run up $50,000 in bills which he could not pay. It is very easy to find cases of catastrophic illness with very large medical bills which the patient cannot pay. Well, if this country had catastrophic insurance, you would end these horror stories, because catastrophic insurance would take care of that tiny percentage of the population which has the bad luck to contract terrible ailments and to run up these bills. But the left wants the horror stories because its ultimate objective is the socialization of American medicine.

Now why does the right oppose catastrophic insurance? The reason is that the right is fundamentally pessimistic. The right argues that a small program of catastrophic insurance will eventually lead to a nationalized health care system. This, they reason, would result because congress would start out with a $10,000 catastrophic health insurance program—that is, the insurance would pay for anything over $10,000—but Congress would not stop there. If it starts at $10,000 now, it will lower the limit to $9,000 next year, $8,000 the year after that, $7,000 the year after that, and pretty soon we would have complete health insurance and complete "free" medicine. I am not particularly interested in the political position of either the right or the left. But I am interested in doing something about the financial tragedy of too many families facing terrible illness that runs up bills which overwhelm them. Catastrophic health insurance would solve this problem. Moreover, it would not be very expensive because, very fortunately in this large country, only a very small percentage of the population is affected by catastrophic illness.

Finally, let me speak to a few additional misconceptions people have about medical care and systems of delivery. First of all, there are no utopias; regardless of the medical system, everybody dies. If you have the notion that by some change in the medical system you are suddenly going to get immortality and have radiant good health forever, you are simply wrong. I have already observed at first hand the medical systems in the Soviet Union, Sweden, Britain, and Israel. The interesting thing to me is that in all of those countries, where medicine is essentially totally socialized, everybody complains all of the time. I am convinced that there are no utopias.

Secondly, if you have a serious illness, it is going to be very expensive because of the nature of medical technology. There is no cheap way of giving a person a kidney or a heart transplant, kidney dialysis, or any one of the many modern procedures. And thirdly, the notion that doctors have some hidden secret weapon of preventive medicine that will guarantee us good health is most oversold. Unfortunately, this notion just is not true. If you believe this assertion, take notice that doctors also get sick and doctors also die. My own view is that prospects of achieving great preventive medicine simply by making some revolutionary changes in the medical care system in this country are just nonsense. The best preventive medicine can be practiced by all of us. If all of us would only stop smoking cigarettes, stop mainlining heroin and other drugs, if we did not overeat, and if we exercised regularly, we would presumably have better health. Unfortunately, most of us do not want to do these things. One of the most important events that has happened for American health recently is the gasoline shortage. The data reveals that in the single month of December, 1,000 fewer people died than a year ago. The reason is that there was less automobile driving. I contend that, indeed, the greatest gains in preventive medicine have nothing to do with the medical care system, per se.

In conclusion, I am arguing in essence that we have a medical care system which has a great many virtues. It works well for most of the population most of the time, and it is admired by other nations of the world. Anyone who argues that revolutionary changes in our medical system are needed, has to bear the burden of proof that his revolutionary changes will not make things worse rather than better. This is not to say that our system is perfect. There are definite weaknesses which must be repaired, and I have made a number of suggestions for correcting these deficiencies. But I emphasize that this so-called "nonsystem" ought to be cherished for how well it really does work. When we are dealing with something as complex, as big, and as intimate as the medical system, it is best to make haste slowly. Evolution rather than revolution is what I suggest for American medicine.

HEALTH SERVICE RESEARCH, HEALTH POLICY, AND THE REAL WORLD

GERALD ROSENTHAL

Introduction

Policy and research are words that conjure up visions of important things. But in discussions about them, we often forget what they really mean. It is some of those things that I want to talk about. This is not, I think, an economist's lecture, except that the fellow who is giving it is an economist. The viewpoints offered here benefit from what happens on the way toward acquiring that expertise. However, it is also the offering of someone who has been a student and in some ways a practitioner of medical care for many years. I have watched our society begin to come to grips with what it perceives to be some of the problems surrounding the delivery of health services. I believe we are backing into new policy decisions without stopping to evaluate the results of past policy decisions. In this context I want to pause and to raise a few issues.

The order of the title of this talk is really wrong. The real world, of course, comes first. Indeed, no matter how we model it, reconstruct it, describe it, in pieces or in Utopian dimensions, the bench mark must always be the real world, its evolution, and its adaptation to the demands and new desires that society imposes on that reality. It is in this context that one must begin to raise questions like, "What do we mean by policy?" "What is health policy, in particular?" and "What does the way we answer that question imply about the issues and the strategies that we use to attempt to change the world?"

I would like first to address that issue in a general way and then to examine some specifics. First, what do you mean by health care policy, and what goals does society seem to possess with respect to the health care system? I will try to describe these goals as the conventional wisdom chooses to articulate them and see if that yields anything useful. I will then

29

talk about the issue in a theoretical way, analyzing the forms that policy can take and the problems that might arise in the policy-making process.

When I have laid out a number of general dilemmas and problems I will discuss two major areas of contemporary health policy. One is the Health Maintenance Organization Bill, which has recently been passed. I will talk about some of the things we should have learned before we passed this bill that we did not learn and some of the things that we had really better learn, having passed it, which we may not learn. The second policy area I will discuss is the issue of National Health Insurance and health insurance strategies generally. This subject has received a great deal of attention, and yet the discussion surrounding it has been very confused. All too often it has got bogged down in arguments over definition. I think that, in policy discussion particularly, the *right* definition is often much less important than the need to understand what it is we are discussing.

For example, someone once asked me, "Are you for national health insurance?" I answered, "How can you be for or against national health insurance? You tell me what you do not like about the medical care system, and I will show you a national health insurance strategy that will make it worse and another one that will make it better." You cannot ask a generic question about what is not a really generalizable issue. In my discussion of national health insurance I really want to talk about what is implicit in the insurance strategy that might achieve our objectives for health service delivery.

Then having opened up these two policy areas, I will raise issues without necessarily resolving them. I want to put the policy choice into a certain context, and then describe what I think is a major issue that we must deal with before the policy discussion can progress beyond the point of tinkering. Again, I will restate: one ought to be clear about one's goals. For tonight, my policy strategy is my presentation, and my goal is really to stimulate and perhaps to stretch the perspective that you come here with about these issues. I do not intend to solve the problems. If I had the answer to all of these questions, I would be either terribly rich or terribly unpopular!

Why a Public Policy?

Let us start with a few words about the goals of public health care policy. It is important to say why we need a public policy at all. There is no reason *ipso facto* to have one. It is clear that the fact that there is a public policy is an evolutionary response to a set of preconceptions reflecting various points of system influence. The government, the people, the states, the profession, all want to influence the medical care system. In some sense, the goals that people hold with regard to the system will not be served in the absence of some kind of intervention in the way that the system is preceding or developing or in the direction it is failing to take.

Essentially, the fact that there is public policy stems directly from the idea that people have, and are entitled to have, a set of collective expectations about the way a certain set of resource-using activities are being utilized. The medical care system is one such activity about which people have very strong collective expectations, and these have been codified in a mythology that asserts that the ability to pay will not constrain access to services, that altruism is required of a physician so that no patient will be turned away, that the effectiveness of technology must be translated into service delivery, and finally, that health care is a right. Many beliefs which one, some, or all of us accept about health care do not emanate from anything except our perception of this set of activities as being more than a matter of private concern between buyers and sellers. If we did not feel this way about medical care, our task would be simple: some people would get it and some people would not get it. If we viewed medical care as a good that provides only personal satisfaction to the user or requires only individual decision making, then there would be no need to have a public policy, particularly regarding the distribution of such services.

There are fancy economic ways to address this issue. One can argue that the consumption and utilization of medical care services exhibit characteristics of significant externalities, that there are external benefits generated in the consumption of such services, and that there are external costs imposed on society by the absence of such utilization. These externalities may be real costs and benefits or simply perceived costs and benefits. That is, I may impose a kind of benefit on society by getting the society to say that, as a matter of principle, people should have access to health services. I may also assert there is a negative impact on a society when such services are unavailable and inaccessible to individuals. Whether these assertions are true or not, if the society really believes them then the asserted externalities become real. The federal government last year spent over $25 billion on health care. We, as a society, passed Medicare and Medicaid and are now considering passage of national health insurance, which is, of course, going to increase government expenditures. It seems clear that society, in general, is willing to exact significant costs for services, even when a good economist can demonstrate that economically many individuals in that society probably would do better to self-insure and take their chances in the market.

It is the existence of externalities that generates the grounds for public policy. But I am taking a broad, rather than a narrow, view of externalities. For my economist friends, Musgrave's argument about "merit wants" is the view of externalities which I suggest is appropriate.[1] That is, there are some things that people have a right to have because society says that they have a right to have it. All people ought to be served even if the people are not able or willing to buy it themselves. Society after all imposes its own worth on itself and therefore ought to be subject to those values. Society is not whimsical. If it were, sociologists, economists, anthropologists, and behavioral scientists would be out of business. These "sciences" exist only because they believe there is order in the chaos that we perceive, and each of us sifts out our own preconception and peddles it as if it were the truth. Because the world is so complicated, we may all be right. But as yet, we have not figured out how to put it together so that you can look at more than one perspective at a time and make sense.

Goals of Health Care Policy

Now, we have to look at the question, What do we mean by the goals of health care policy? If you look at the literature in medical care, it is clear that we have chosen to define these goals in terms of properties of the system—that medical services be accessible, available, and of high quality. All of these goals get codified around a peculiar articulation of the public policy position—i.e., that health care is a right. This ennunciation makes health care the ultimate Musgravian merit want.

The right to health

From a legal standpoint, what does it mean for something to be a right? Does that imply that there is a general objective in society to get to a point where people have a ready access to good health care services, or does it mean that society is incurring a kind of contractual obligation? We have some experience with this issue. Within the last few years, suits against a number of states have been brought on behalf of parents of mentally retarded children to force the states to meet their obligation to educate those children. The right to education is an obligation. It is a contractual obligation of the state. There is no ambiguity about it at all. The state must make available to the children in the state such educational facilities as are adequate to meet some minimum standard of educational perfor-

---

1. A merit want involves a good or service that society considers so meritorious that it is willing to augment the private market's production of that good or service through public subsidies or public production. Free public education and subsidized higher education are examples of merit wants. For further discussion of this point see Richard A. Musgrave, *The Theory of Public Finance* (New York: McGraw-Hill, 1959), pp. 13-14.—Ed.

mance. A number of cases have been heard this year, and the courts have ruled in favor of the plaintiffs.

Now what is the right to health? It is important to realize that, unlike education, health is not something anyone can give you, so there is some legalistic ambiguity. If it is a right to medical services, it would be a little more comforting and more plausible. But what does it mean to say that people have a right to health or that health care is a right? In what sense is it a right? That remains an unresolved issue, but its assertion does at least legitimize the public involvement. The form that this right takes is in terms of medical care services. Operationally, it constitutes striving for accessibility, availability, and high-quality services for all people.

Basic forms of policy and conditions for policy making

Let me talk now about the generic forms which policy can take. These are the reasons for having public policy. That is, if a system behaves in a certain way, it produces a certain end result, but if we want those end results to be different we identify the needs of the system by saying that the system does not have certain properties, which in fact we would like it to have. Policies, in my view, have got to be seen basically as interventions in the system of service delivery. That is, they are impositions from outside. For instance, on the one hand, a practicing physician might try to do things a little differently because he thinks it might work better or it might be more effective. Such an individual decision is not policy, it is just somebody going about his business. On the other hand, when I stand outside the system and decide to fund a pilot project in a certain area, that decision is an intervention. I am buying somebody into behavior that they would not otherwise undertake, and I do not deliver any services.

Basically, policies require two things simultaneously. One is some preconception of an inadequacy in the system. The other is the recognition of an opportunity for change. It is not enough to say the system does badly. To form a policy, somebody must say, "If you do the following, you are likely to make the system work better." Research plays an important role here because it can analyze this cause-effect relationship.

There are four basic forms of policy, all of which are really points on a continuum of types of policy. At one extreme are *prohibitive* strategies. These policies arise when it is both within the authority of the policy maker and possible to preclude certain forms of behavior. An example is that no one who is not a physician shall prescribe drugs. Other examples could be offered. A second type of policy restricts behavior. The policy maker says that anybody can go into the business of caring for the elderly, but if you want to call yourself a nursing home and get reimbursed for your services, you are going to have to do certain kinds of things. *Restrictive* policy is a little softer than a prohibition. On the other side, we have what I call *stimulative* policies. We provide incentives for certain kinds of behavior. Hill-Burton grants for the development of hospital facilities are one example. Student scholarships or fellowships are another. As a last type, some policies are *coercive* in that they require certain behavior.

Certain properties of policy making also seem to hold generally true. Prohibitive or coercive policies must be based on a great deal of certainty, since what you propose in making them is definitely what will happen; they have to be right, otherwise you make the system worse. For a stimulative or a restrictive strategy, on the other hand, you do not have to be that sure. You just make it a little more likely that what you want to happen will happen. If the system really does not want it to happen, it will not happen. That is perfectly all right. After all, how far wrong can you go? In other fields, they call that reducing your downside risk, which probably has some value for social policy making.

Another point that comes out of an analysis of general policy behavior is the notion that if you really have conflicting goals, then you must sacrifice one goal in order to achieve another. In health care policy, if you aim for high-quality services you have to give up some availability. The very elegant arguments of Jan Tinbergen make it clear that no single policy can best serve two nonidentical goals.[2] More operationally, society recognizes a specific problem in the system. It analyzes that problem and discovers one vehicle that seems to solve the problem. So a policy is formed and implemented. The trouble is that this specific policy is likely to impinge in lots of different ways on the rest of the system about which you have some feelings, and with respect to which you have some goals. In this general setting it becomes very hard to make appropriate policy.

Moreover, you have to impose on any problem another issue, one which is often ignored—that is, that the fundamental economic dilemma of choice emerges in the area of policy just as in any other. In other words, you really do have scarcity in spite of the "affluent society" and the inaccurately labelled Galbraithean ethic. The notion that there is not scarcity is ludicrous. And yet, we have really often dealt with policy in the health care field as if every strategy were additive; that is, as if every deficiency could be cured by additional resources. On the false assumption that strategies are not competitive, we have ignored a number of significant trade-offs that must inevitably occur in areas where resources are truly scarce.

2. In *On the Theory of Economic Policy* (Amsterdam: North Holland, 1952), chap. 7.

Quality-quantity trade-off

An area of trade-off which is central to health care policy and which not only has colored the choices that we have made for the last decade or two but has implications for the way we might make subsequent choices is the important trade-off between quantity and quality. Quality imposes resource uses, and therefore one incurs costs in order to achieve a certain quality. When you try to achieve the goals previously mentioned, accessibility and equity of distribution, and also continually emphasize quality requirements, you have a dynamic that says that one must look at the system's inherent prejudices. Are there biases built into the system which make it likely that, when resources are added to the system, they will move toward one goal rather than the other? To me, the experience of the last fifteen years makes it obvious that quality wins. The dynamic in the system is always conducive to improving the quality of services for those who are already in the system of medical services at the expense of expanding access for those who are not in the system. The whole literature of consumer participation is deficient in this respect. It views as "consumers" only those who are already participating in the system and it does not treat the problem of the people who are not in the system.

Now, how does this bias become articulated? The regional medical program—the former heart disease, cancer, stroke program—was predicated heavily on the idea that although we know technologically how to do many things we do not get the services out to the people. So the policy makers went to service delivery settings that were already points of access for people, and added coronary care units, intensive care units, and continuing education. Obviously, this policy intensified the quality of services available to the people who were in the system. There are some exceptions to this effect. Regions did begin to build networks of emergency services, but unfortunately emergency services, the bastard child of the health care world anyway, were not central to the program.

The arguments for a bias toward technological improvement are also supported by the dynamics of malpractice. In order to demonstrate that you have practiced adequately, you have to show that you have covered yourself. How do you cover yourself? Well, if somebody invented a new test for a certain disease and a patient has any of the symptoms, the physician feels that he had better run the test. This is another instance of the way in which the resources available to the system are co-opted to impose more and more services on those who are already in the system while the option of letting in people who are outside the system remains unexplored.

There is another reason why the medical care system stresses quality over quantity. This is the fact that the whole training of physicians and the whole science of medicine is built on a view that *need* is a binary characteristic, you either need medical care or you don't. That is, if something is potentially technologically relevant to your symptomatic state, applying it in your case is good medicine. Consequently fame and fortune is often gained by developing new ways of dealing with old things. All of the technological change in the industry has really been directed at quality enhancement. Nobody says, "We do a fair job at this kind of thing. I don't want to do it any better. I want to find out how to make it cheaper. When you find out how to do it for half the resources, then I am going to use the same amount of total resources, but I am going to go over to that town down there that does not have any medical services, open a clinic and do it cheap there, too." I repeat, nobody takes this position. And in contrast, improving quality is easy and unambiguous. Furthermore, it does not require any explicit specifications of the benefits. *That it is better is quite sufficient.*

Now, if you believe that the resources you are dealing with are not scarce, then this view is correct. But we are dealing with scarcity, and the issue is really one of distribution.

Role of research

Where does research come into all of this? Research has a number of roles in the policy area. For one, let's start from a policy, any policy—National Health Insurance, HMOs, Comprehensive Health Planning Act, it does not really matter which one. Research, or what we call research, becomes a vehicle for testing the assumptions of the policy. Two key questions are: What is it that the policy really said it was going to do? and ,Did it really do it? Now, one can ask, why should that be done after the fact? Because you cannot always tell before the fact and we have been wrong too many times. It turns out that we do this type of research under the guise of evaluation. Yet, it really is research. Since we rarely set down the objectives in the first place, it is very hard to tell what evaluation is.

The second role of research in policy is to identify the costs and the benefits of strategies. We no longer are free of the burden of articulating the costs and the benefits. We must at least attempt to identify a good strategy by comparing costs and benefits of alternatives.

Let me give you an example of what I mean. The State of California presented data that indicated it cost $5,000 per case to discover and treat a child with Phenylketonuria (PKU). Since many PKU children will end up mentally retarded and it costs the state $5,000 per year per mentally retarded individual, whose average stay in a mental institution is twenty-five years, the state figured that they saved $125,000 a child for a $5,000 expenditure. In reviewing the state's analysis, I asked how many babies they had to test before they found a case. The answer was 16,000-18,000. I then asked what the tests cost. The answer was that this expenditure was not in the state budget; rather, they billed that to individual parents. Since the lab charges average $2.50—that's $40,000 per identified child for the lab tests alone to find a case of this disease. And yet, this cost was not counted in the calculation. Why? Because the state did not pay for the tests.

On the benefit side, I then noted that PKU patients in California mental institutions accounted for only about 1 percent of the inpatient population. Why did they believe they would reduce the cost of operating mental institutions by 1 percent if they reduced patients by 1 percent? More likely, it would save about 1 percent of the cost of meals, not $5,000 a year. More generally, the hospital business has been "average-costed" to death. There is a myth here. In fact, when you reduce your inpatient occupancy by 10 percent you are not going to reduce your cost 10 percent. Hospitals are typically staffed for capacity and how many patients are in or out on any given date makes little difference to the total operating cost of the hospital.

The independent researcher has an obligation to do an objective analysis of costs and benefits. Such an analysis will generate some policy options. The researcher ought to identify different strategies that one might wish to utilize in order to change the system in certain ways. It is not up to the analyst to decide whether the result is better. Rather, the point is that knowing how the system works and how it behaves helps the policy maker select an intervention to make it different.

Some Examples of Policy

Health Maintenance Organization bill

Let us now take two recent examples of policy decisions and attempt to trace through what I infer have been the stimuli for them and the focuses of thinking around them.

One example is the Health Maintenance Organization bill, an intriguing piece of legislation, which has recently been passed by Congress. It provides resources to stimulate the development of what are known as Health Maintenance Organizations. These organizations, often prepaid group plans, contract to provide a comprehensive set of services to an identified population on a capitation payment basis. This bill comes, I think, not from a desire to make service more available to the population, but rather reflects another policy objective which is prominent in the public view, namely the policy referred to euphemistically as cost containment. Over many years we have identified a number of prepaid group practices which tend to use hospital services a lot less than do other settings. That is, given two populations with identical characteristics, the one served by a prepaid group practice will have hospitalization rates significantly lower than the one served by a fee-for-service solo practice. Therefore, it is argued, prepaid groups are able to provide similar benefits for lower cost. Partly on the basis of evidence, the Congress decided to support prepaid group practice through the HMO legislation.

The background of this bill is enlightening. The first point that was raised as a real issue was the discovery that, while the federal government had been supporting the principles of prepaid group practice for many years and although it was a large payer for services under Medicare, it could not prepay group practices for their services. It could only pay on a fee-for-service basis, since Medicare reimburses only for units of service delivered. It was suggested that a Part C be added to Medicare which would say that, when there was a Health Maintenance Organization (HMO) that would contract to provide to an identified set of the covered population a package of benefits at least equal to the Medicare benefits, then the Medicare program would prepay an amount up to 95 percent of the average expenses per Medicare beneficiary in the area on behalf of that individual. The view was that if we were in favor of prepaid group practice we ought to at least be willing to pay for Medicare recipients through that means as well as any other. Although this bill never went anywhere, the phrase HMO found a lot of friends.

One result was the Health Maintenance Organization bill which essentially provides grants-in-aid and start-up money for such settings and prescribes a set of benefits which eligible HMOs must provide.

By this bill, Congress is trying to influence both quality and quantity of medical care. The legislators knew of the good experience with ambulatory care offsetting hospital care and cost reduction in HMOs. However, they also tried to incorporate another element of conventional wisdom, namely that the only good care is comprehensive full medical care. Remember what I said about quality enhancement at the expense of access? You cannot often have both, and you will most likely get more quality. My cheapest estimate of what it would cost an HMO to provide the stipulated set of benefits in the required way is approximately $1300 or $1400 a year per family. This estimate is far above the most expensive group plans presently in existence, which average about $700-$800/year per family. Moreover, the cost containment experience of present-day HMOs is closely tied to the fact that they do not provide comprehensive services on demand to all. They provide from the most important to the least important until they run out of money, and then they do not provide any more services. For example, we all believe that everyone needs an annual physical. If you go to many prepaid groups there is a long waiting period for a physical exam, particularly for people in their 20s and 30s. Why? Because the staff handles emergencies; they must do dangerous difficult things; they must handle acute episodes, and annual physicals have the lowest priority. After all, you can not do everything—for $680 a year. In addition, I, for one, am not willing to spend $1500 a year for everything. I'm prepared to take my chances and not do a few things. In sum then, Congress generalized an HMO experience, then threw in another kind of objective, and ended up with a policy that may be nonviable.

Now, what can the responses be? Well, they can subvert the standards, which would not be so bad. By the way, *subvert* is not meant in a perjorative sense. You can use another word: *substitute, modify, adapt, realisticalize,* or whatever. Or they can increase the start-up money so that somebody will take them up on their offer and run a subsidized, high quality, first-class pilot demonstration project. Then later we will see what we can generalize from this demonstration.

National health insurance

Now let us turn to national health insurance. What is it? As all insurance is, it's a response to the economic uncertainty generated by some possibility of financially adverse happenstance. Essentially, insurance only deals with economic risks. It says that under certain kinds of circumstances, it provides you with money. And it says that it can only deal with those dimensions of the circumstance that have to do with your incurring economic loss. That is what all insurance is supposed to do. It does not deliver any services, and it does not provide any services. It is not a supply strategy. An insurance policy says that there is some probability that something will happen to you that will cost you a lot of money. If you pay so much money in advance, you can buy certainty in the form of a limitation of that potential loss.

When Congress was developing the Medicare legislation, it heard testimony about how old people were not able to get services because they had low incomes. In 1964, when the bill was under discussion, I argued that there would be significant supply pressures generated by the passage of the Medicare legislation. I made the argument that we ought to take the Hill-Burton funds and change the allocation scheme so that those areas which would feel the greatest impact on supply from the Medicare-generated demand would be able to draw on those funds for expansion of facilities. That struck me as a logical thing to do. I did not know then that logic was not really a criterion for policy making. The answer I got, from economists I might add, was that such potential supply constraints would take care of themselves. Yet, I kept asking, how could one support a piece of legislation to get people in the market for services and not attempt to assure the availability of the services? The Medicare strategy was to let these people have an "even shake" in the marketplace. In effect it said, "I am going to pay your bill so just go out there and get those services. Of course if you don't get them that is not my problem, because I do not deliver any services."

We said at the beginning of this discussion that the market will allocate in an efficient way only if no one else cares about your transactions. But we have already established that this condition is not present in this case, because of externalities. The point is, we want to use the market as an allocation scheme, but we say that the market really will not allocate right because many of the aged will not have enough money. Since we want them to get needed health services in that market, we will bankroll them into the system. Unfortunately, we discovered that this method costs a lot of money. At this point the cost containment objective rears its ugly head.

We have numerous strategies to contain costs. One is to make the people (elderly) put up some of the money. So we set, or increase, what is called a deductible. You must spend the first $50, say, before we will pay. And then we say that you must share some of the total cost for medical services. This we call co-insurance. We pay 80 percent and you pay 20 percent. As a result, we have reduced what is coming out of the public coffer. So we have done two things at once: offset the poorly made market allocation by increasing the elderly's ability to pay and then constrained the costs of the program by making the recipients pay some of the cost themselves. But what has really happened? We had a policy that wanted to reallocate services to the needy. And yet, the cost containment response is to move back to the market allocation, at a reduced price, mind you, but still back to the market allocation.

The same thing has happened to Medicaid in many states. You cannot change the benefit package, but you certainly can redefine eligibility. If the cost is too large, you just cut some people out. In this way, you get the pool of potential eligibles down to where it stays within the state budgetary requirement. In sum then, if you use a strategy for the equity objective, as the insurance plan really started out to be by getting the insured a "fairer" share of the market, and then use the market allocation strategies as a cost containment device, you have something that is at best inefficient.

Now Congress is talking about national health insurance and there everybody is cagey. The Health Security Act includes everything in the medical care market. It will have area groups to allocate supply, quality control, and the insurance mechanism. Most of all, everybody is going to get all the services, i.e., comprehensive, high-quality, full-fledged medical services. Experience suggests "you can't get there from here." It's a snare and a deception to say that we can have it all. What will really happen is that some of the people are going to get it all and the rest of the people will get very little. You are not providing any viable alternative.

Alternative Approaches to Policy

Now how do you find a viable alternative? Let me suggest there are certain areas where we need do some serious research. We have skirted the issue of quality of care for years and I think we have reached the end of our string. The Bureau of Health Services Research will put $6 million into quality-assurance research in the next six or eight months. The commitment is widely shared by enough people at HEW and in the Congress for them to spend the money to find out what quality means. It is essential to distinguish between one type of quality and another type of quality. Until we get to a point where we can distinguish between *this* "better" and another "better," we are never going to understand the trade-offs. In that case, the system's inherent bias toward enhancing what it already does will always prevail. The cost containment perspective is wrong because the cost that the government is looking at in that strategy is exactly like the cost that the State of California looked at in saying that to find a PKU case it cost $5,000/child rather than $45,000 or maybe $140,000. The typical rule says that if the government does not pay it then it is not relevant to policy. For the public to take that perspective is myopia of the highest order. *We* pay it either way.

We do have to be able to articulate the choices in such a way that others can help make them. We have to be able to serve the people. To say that "health care is a right" means that, given the resources that go into health services, certain distributional properties will prevail. The government could make the right to health care operational by guaranteeing some *minimum adequate service* after which the individual is on his own. When we were ready to put more resources into the medical care system, then we could raise the floor.

One of the problems with this approach to equity, however, is that we have always described our health care system in terms of the *best* that it can do rather than the *worst* that it does. If you take a thousand people at random in this country and evaluate their experiences with the receiving and utilization of health services in the last year, you are going to get a mixed bag, ranging from the magnificent to the appalling. *If equity is a real objective of society, then treating an expansion of the magnificent and an improvement in the appalling as equally desirable is just not acceptable social policy.* Alternatively, you can say that you do not care and get out of the policy analysis business in the health field. If you want to leave it up to where people put their dollars, then just sit back and accept the market results. But when we assert the legitimacy of the so-called right to health, at that point it becomes obligatory to do something.

Unfortunately, it turns out that we have a technological problem. Nobody can describe what a *minimum adequate level* of service is without being ambiguous. They can tell me what is in a comprehensive, high quality medical care service package, but they cannot tell me what a minimum adequate level is.

Now my guess is that we have gone about policy making in a backwards way. An early major area of public policy in health care was an insurance approach stressing economic protection. We started with the relatively trivial but expensive. We did not start where people encountered the system. We started with what happens with people who are in the system who get to the point where they are in the hospital and they cannot pay their bills. And so we have emphasized insurance.

We did not face the issue of getting everybody into the system. Suppose we had said we would give everybody two visits to a physician a year and after that they were on their own. If we had done that twenty years ago, we would be years ahead, because we would know something about what is coming into the system and what is going on. We would also have a basis for a need-oriented allocation because then a physician could look at the people who come to him and decide, for example, that for 30 percent it is not important to go any further, for 20 percent medical facilities to send them to are desperately needed. He doesn't need facilities enough for 50 percent of them, however, only for 30 percent.

Instead, we have planned the whole system backwards. We talk about systems organized around a hospital, when indeed the hospital is a back-up support service for a whole variety of face-to-face contacts with patients who much more frequently need ambulatory services. Then we try policies that look as if we are turning it around, except every time "push comes to shove" we revert to one of two positions: either we let the market do it, because we feel that it is too complicated and we do not really know what medical need is after all, or we do the best we can with what we have, and that always means that we are going to put more money in the system where our money has already gone.

The use of minimum standards in policy decisions is prevalent in other areas. For example, we do not tell people they cannot buy better education, but we do maintain a public education system that establishes a kind of floor. We also, believe it or not, are assured a certain quality of bread—although the level at which we guarantee it, while nutritionally sound, is sort of boring. In other areas of public policy we assert that we maintain a minimum floor, but we really do not. For example, in transportation we have taken the opposite route. What we really should have done is to have built good public transportation and allowed people who wanted to own cars to do so. What we did instead was accept the idea that people wanted to have cars and conclude that it was not necessary to build a good public transportation system.

Conclusion

Now let me reiterate my main argument. I said I would talk to some extent on health research, health policy, and the real world, and I said that title was really backwards. We are talking about the real world. Health policy is kind of an intervention in that world, attempting to modify its behavior and performance. In the health area, the intervention is needed because we do share widely a sense that medical care is a service whose distribution we care about, and it is our concern that, because of the degree of interaction in the marketplace, the market solution will not be the right one by definition. Economists would agree that, if a good or service displays significant externalities, the market solution will be suboptimal. And indeed that turns out to be true.

I have tried to describe a couple of areas of general strategy where the policies, based upon a certain knowledge about the world, really tended to conflict with espoused objectives. In the case of HMOs, we do not know what to do yet. We are still in the process of developing policy. In the health insurance strategy we have a track record. Every time we have got into escalation on the demand side and really discovered how much it cost, mainly because of the constraints on the supply side, we have moved back to a market allocation strategy through deductibles and co-insurance, or, at the ultimate, through considering simply a catastrophic coverage and none of the early coverage at all. The latter approach says that you are all on your own in the marketplace, but if total economic disaster strikes big brother will bail you out.

One of the points that I have tried to emphasize has to do with health care as a right and what it takes to make that right operational. I have argued that in order to do that you must move away from the quality enhancement bias relative to equity objectives. This requires the development of a technological means of defining *minimum adequate levels* of care. We must define the floor, because we are never going to make a viable guarantee for the peak. We could operationalize a social contract that essentially obligates a floor if we could agree on what the floor was. My argument is simply that any floor which was based on ambulatory care would be a good place to start because that strategy will generate information. We are presently tinkering all over the place. It would be very hard to share with you my sense of frustration at the numbers of people who are running around worrying about these problems and tinkering, concocting, and contriving solutions to them. The research community is supposed to be the referee and monitor in that game. I do believe that a technological move in the direction of specifying the floor for performance by a medical care system would be quite useful from a policy standpoint. Clearly, one of our problems is that the policy objective has not been viably identified. Yet, I think, a policy focused on the floor is consistent with the social dynamic and also is one whose cost is containable.

Well, I have no grand finale. My intention was to provoke, to stimulate, get you to view policy making from a perspective of what is involved, and to share with you some of my close-to-the-surface feelings about its problems. It seems to me that people have a high level of expectations with regard to health services and that there is a fairly widespread feeling that somehow we really do not make the grade.

Furthermore, what was for a while thought of as a poor people's problem is now seen as a general problem. If you go to people in any income class, in any city, and ask them what they view as the difficulties of health services, they talk about the same things. The services are hard to get to; there is a high degree of uncertainty of access; they do not really know how to deal with the system. They lack the security of knowing how the system will deal with them and what is happening to them. Moreover, they feel victimized by the medical system and always have a tremendous fear of cost and expense.

What I am suggesting is that, by starting to deal only with the fear of cost, we are going to get in a corner where we are merely narrowing that fear to the lower end of the income scale again (probably not the very poor for whom separate appropriations will be made) and buying off the middle. That will take the heat out of demands for radical change in the system. A lot of people have said that if the collective bargaining movement in this country had not been so successful in developing health programs after World War II we would have had national health insurance ten years ago. I suspect that is true. There is a kind of diffusion of impact that reduces the politically critical mass.

Moreover, it does seem to me that medical care is not the biggest problem that people have in their lives. It is high on everybody's list, but it is not at the top of anybody's list. If you talk to the poor, the problem is education and employment. To the middle class, we must deal with higher prices, crime, education, and then health. Therefore, medical care is not the hottest issue politically. I feel that things are going to happen with health care because the nation's leaders have decided that it is an issue that has come of age. Unfortunately, we have not really faced up to the specifics about what we are trying to do and therefore have skirted much of the problem. HMOs and NHI are two of the newest steps in the tinkering. While we are making some better policies than we did in the past, we have not dealt with the quality issue, the *peak versus floor* dynamic. Until we do that, we are a long way from home.

AN ECONOMIC ANALYSIS OF THE
MARKET FOR NURSES

DONALD E. YETT

I would like to talk about some material contained in my forthcoming book "An Economic Analysis of Nurse Supply and Demand." It was prepared under the auspices of the U.S. Public Health Service (Bureau of Health Resources Development, Division of Nursing), and it will be two years next month since the final draft was submitted to the sponsor for publication. During this time we have been engaged in a dispute concerning the sponsor's desire to delete certain sections from the manuscript before it is published.[1]

I believe that the material in these sections should be made public, and, therefore, I have decided to try to summarize it for you here. Indeed, it is possible—but I hope not too likely—that the members of this audience will be the only people who will know about some of the major conclusions of my study. When I finish presenting this material you will probably wonder why it is considered so sensitive that the sponsors feel it must be removed before my book can be published. The points I have to make are

---

1. On 30 April 1974 (subsequent to the date of this talk) the Director of the Bureau of Health Resources Development wrote, in his words, to "confirm my agreement to remove the restrictions on publication of your analyses and interpretation of the data resulting from this study with the provision that a statement be inserted in a prominent place in any such publication to the effect that the analyses, interpretations and discussions are those of the author and do not necessarily represent the position of the U.S. Government on such matters. HEW retains the right to publish or otherwise use data from this study in whatever manner it sees fit to carry out the purpose of its program. It is my understanding that you concur with this arrangement and that you will go ahead now and seek to have your analyses published in the private press." On the same date, I entered into a contract with D. C. Heath and Company for the publication of the book later this year under the title "An Economic Analysis of the Nurse Shortage."

Full documentation of all of the material in my talk will be contained in the forthcoming book. Except for citations to direct quotations, I have dispensed with the usual footnote references in this presentation.

hardly sensational or inflammatory. Nevertheless, I hope that they will help to stimulate a reconsideration of the existing program of federal subsidies for nurse training.

The market for professional nurses is a fascinating and important topic for economic analysis. Its participants on the supply side constitute the largest health manpower occupation requiring formal training and licensing. Over 95 percent of the practitioners are female, which makes this the largest almost exclusively female occupation other than domestic self-employment. Nurses produce a service which is often described as a necessity rather than a want and which many public health authorities believe has been in short supply for 35 or 40 years. Considering the sense of urgency attached to the so-called shortage of nurses, it is not surprising that Congress initiated a massive nurse-training subsidy program in 1964 and authorized expenditures of approximately 1.3 billion dollars under this program over the past ten years. A short time later, in a totally unrelated move, Congress enacted the Medicare and Medicaid programs (Titles XVIII and XIX of the Social Security Act). Although the purpose of these programs was to provide adequate health care to the elderly and indigent, they also had the effect of further increasing the demand for nurses.

Economic characteristics

Before turning attention to the nurse-training subsidy program, which is the heart of what I want to talk with you about tonight, I would like to review briefly the economic characteristics of the market for nurses. It is important to understand the salient features of the unique market as background for interpreting the pros and cons of the federal program designed to greatly expand the supply of nurses.

Most nurses are either secondary wage earners, or they plan to be in the near future. As a result, they exhibit very low levels of wage-induced geographic mobility. This fact, combined with the site-specific nature of the service they produce, means that local area nurse markets have a high degree of autonomy. That is, conditions in other areas will have little effect on the behavior of either nurses or employers in a given locality.

Hospitals account for about 70 percent of total nurse employment, and thus they constitute the dominant employers in virtually all local nurse markets. Indeed, their influence is so pervasive that most nurse markets can best be characterized in terms of the degree of employer competition in the hospital sector. Hospitals in rural areas are often monopsonistic nurse employers. Those in other areas are oligopsonistic. In communities with a small number of hospitals, oligopsonistic wage policies require no formal coordination. And large urban areas almost universally have hospital associations, which, among other things, operate what they call "wage standardization" programs. The existence of these programs confirms the members' belief that, if they acted individually, each would have a noticeable effect on nurses' salaries. Because of this belief, they voluntarily join together to avoid what they fear would be costly wage wars, which would have little overall effect after they were over on total nurse employment.

The fact that urban hospitals adhere to association wage recommendations, even in the absence of effective enforcement mechanisms, strongly suggests that each believes it faces a rather steep nurse supply curve. Numerous independent estimates of the elasticity in the supply of nurses support this belief. Further support is provided by a recent University of Southern California study which found that less than 2 percent of the job changes that were observed among hospital nurses involved a wage-induced move into or out of the Los Angeles area, despite the continued existence of large nurse wage differentials between Los Angeles and other areas. Moreover, all of the wage-induced mobility flows within the area were extremely small. For example, shifts between hospitals and nonnursing employment were virtually nil. Wage-induced reentry into the nurse labor force was approximately half of a percent. Interarea hospital moves were found to amount to about 3 percent and shifts between hospitals and other types of employment for nurses amounted to 2.3 percent of the total. This is not to say that nurses do not move around a lot. Obviously, they do—as is apparent from their annual turnover rate which averages around 50-60 percent. The important point is that little of this movement is due to wages or related factors.

Faced with supply curves which exhibit significant positive slopes, oligopsonistic and monopsonistic hospital employers report that they want to hire more nurses than they can at existing wage levels. I have called unfilled positions of this sort *equilibrium job vacancies.* They are quite different from unfilled positions arising as a result of dynamic increases in demand relative to supply. The latter—which can be filled given sufficient time for the necessary market adjustments—I call *effective vacancies.* They exist in all fields of nursing, whereas the former are found only in the hospital fields.

Approximately 15 percent of all active nurses are employed as private duty or office nurses. Both of these fields are closely related to hospital nursing. Although private duty nurses are employed directly by their patients, about 98 percent of them perform their services in hospitals. Virtually all private duty employment is arranged through nurse registries, which as a matter of policy set basic eight-hour rates in conformity with the wages of hospital staff nurses. As a result, large numbers of unfilled private duty requests are common. Office nurses are recruited by physicians who, in turn, acquire their knowledge of nurse salaries and working conditions from the time they spend in hospitals. By offering better working conditions and other amenities, physicians find it easy to recruit nurses for their offices at the same salaries paid by the hospitals in their communities. Job vacancies are low and complaints of nurse shortages are nonexistant in the office field.

In general, the remaining fields of nursing are the highest paid. Basically, these are the nurses who work in industries where they constitute only a small percentage of the total work force. In such industries, nurses' salaries are often administratively set on the basis of the wages paid to the majority of the workers in the industry. Thus, for example, industrial nurse wages closely correspond to the wages of production workers in manufacturing. Public health nurses commonly are covered by civil service pay scales. Boards of Education pay school nurses approximately the same salaries as primary and secondary school teachers. And nurse educators are paid salaries comparable to those of other college instructors. Since their wage setting practices result in paying "above scale," at least in relation to hospitals, these employers of nurses face what amount to horizontal supply curves. They could pay lower salaries without encountering any serious "shortages." The fact that they do not pay lower salaries means that the benefits of having few job vacancies (indeed waiting lists are common), low turnover, and long tenure, outweigh the small additional payroll costs involved. As long as this continues to be true, employment practices in these fields will have little or no effect on the general level of nurse salaries, which will follow the trend set by the dominant employers—hospitals.

Federal Programs

With this background in mind, I would now like to discuss the efforts of the federal government to alleviate what is widely believed to be the shortage of nurses. Although there were some earlier federal programs addressed at this problem—e.g., the Cadet Nurse Corps during World War II—the passage of the Nurse Training Act of 1964 (NTA) was the culmination of many years of planning and lobbying by nursing leaders. NTA initiated a five-year $287,630,000 program ($298 million after amendments), which, it was hoped, would lead to a 75 percent increase in the annual number of nursing school graduations by the year 1975. It included authorizations of approximately $90 million in matching funds for school construction and renovation; grants to all types of nursing schools in the amount of $17 million for projects to expand or strengthen their teaching programs; $41 million to nonprofit diploma schools to help offset the costs of additional students expected as a result of the Act; $50 million to continue and expand the nurse traineeship program to prepare graduate nurses as teachers, administrators, supervisors and specialists; and $85 million for low-interest, partially "forgivable" student loans.

Two amendments to NTA were passed in 1966 and one in 1967. The first permitted the transfer of unused construction grant appropriations from one category of school to another (the funds for baccalaureate schools were being exhausted while those for Associate of Arts [AA] and diploma programs were not being fully used). The second amendment established a scholarship program which allowed schools that were able to provide matching funds to award from $200 to $1000 per year to needy students, and it authorized $15 million for this program during the last three years of the Act. The third amendment allowed schools the choice of participating in the student loan program via a revolving fund.

Table 1 compares the actual appropriations and awards (obligations) with the amounts authorized for each major section of the 1964 NTA. In the first year of the program Congress appropriated virtually all of the amounts authorized. However, because of insufficient response, only $788,000 of the $4 million for payments to diploma programs were awarded. The following year only about one-third of the amount authorized was appropriated and awarded for such payments. Again, in fiscal 1967, although appropriations were only 60 percent of authorizations for this program, only half of this amount could be awarded. Finally, in 1968 both appropriations and awards were brought into line with experience. Clearly, the willingness and/or ability of diploma schools to train more nurses in response to such subsidies had been overestimated.

The influence of the 1966 amendment permitting the transfer of unused construction funds between types of programs is also evident. In 1966 awards were only about two-thirds of authorizations and appropriations; but in 1967, after the amendment, all three were nearly equal. Awards lagged in 1968; and appropriations were cut to about one-third of the amount authorized in 1969, when the total awarded exceeded the amount appropriated by the size of the carry-over from 1968. Similarly, the effects of the 1967 amendment permitting schools to participate in the student loan program via revolving funds are also reflected in Table 1. Awards for student loan funds were about one-fourth less than was authorized and appropriated for 1967. However, awards exceeded the amounts appropriated (which, in turn, were substantially below the amounts authorized) in 1968 and 1969. The difference came from the sale of revolving fund participation certificates.

Table 1

Authorization, Appropriations, and Awards under the Provisions of the Nurse Training Act of 1964 and Amendments

(in Thousands of Dollars)

Period (Fiscal Year)	Construction	Special Project Grants	Payments to Diploma Schools	Student Loans	Traineeships	Opportunity Grants	Total
1965							
Authorized	0	2,000	4,000	3,100	8,000	...	17,100
Appropriated	0	2,000	4,000	3,100	8,000	...	17,100
Awarded	0	1,990	788	3,090	7,879	...	13,747
1966							
Authorized	15,000	3,000	7,000	8,900	9,000	...	42,900
Appropriated	15,000	3,000	2,500	8,900	9,000	...	38,400
Awarded	10,539	1,928	2,146	8,871	8,784	...	32,268
1967							
Authorized	25,000	4,000	10,000	16,800	10,000	3,000	68,800
Appropriated	25,000	4,000	6,000	16,900	10,000	500	62,400
Awarded	22,082	3,518	3,069	12,677	9,790	0	51,136
1968							
Authorized	25,000	4,000	10,000	25,300	11,000	5,000	80,300
Appropriated	25,000	4,000	3,000	16,000	10,000	5,000	63,000
Awarded	18,490	3,999	3,000	16,390	9,864	4,120	55,863
1969							
Authorized	25,000	4,000	10,000	30,900	12,000	7,000	88,900
Appropriated	8,000	4,000	3,000	9,610	10,470	6,552	41,632
Awarded	18,060	4,000	3,000	16,008	10,468	6,552	58,088
1965-69							
Authorized	90,000	17,000	41,000	85,000	50,000	15,000	298,000
Appropriated	73,000	17,000	18,500	54,510	47,470	12,052	222,532
Awarded	69,171	15,435	12,003	57,036	46,785	10,672	211,102

With certain modifications, Title II of the Health Manpower Act of 1968 (HMA) extended through fiscal 1971 the same six areas of assistance covered by the 1964 NTA (as amended). One modification involved the requirement that a school have an accredited nurse-training program in order to be eligible for support under most provisions of the 1964 NTA. This condition for participation in the program was objectionable to many schools offering associate degrees in nursing. The bulk of these schools are community colleges, and their administrators did not want to accept a precedent for separate accreditation of each major leading to an A.A. degree. The HMA overcame this problem by making a nurse-training program eligible for support if the educational institution in which it is located is accredited by a regional accrediting body or by a state agency recognized by the state commissioner of education for this purpose. Another modification involved expanding the provision regulating payments to diploma programs to include baccalaureate and associate degree schools as well (i.e., "Payments to Diploma Schools" became "Institutional Grants"). The formula for computing the size of these grants was liberalized, and eligibility requirements were charged. However, as Table 2 shows, these changes had no effect on the programs covered because no funds for such grants were appropriated.

The HMA made any public or nonprofit agency, organization, or institution eligible for special project grants. Moreover, the scope of the grants was enlarged to cover the costs of projects to: (1) plan, develop, or establish new nurse-training programs; (2) support research in the various fields of nursing education; (3) assist schools of nursing which are in serious financial straits to meet their costs of operation; (4) assist schools which need financial assistance to meet accreditation requirements; and (5) assist any eligible agency, organization, or institution to meet the cost of special projects which will help to increase the supply of adequately trained nursing personnel.

Virtually all of the modifications in the student loan program were designed to make it more attractive to a wider range of potential students. They included: (1) giving licensed practical nurses (in addition to first-year students) preference in granting loans; (2) increasing the maximum loan from $1,000 to $1,500 per academic year (up to a maximum total of $6,000); (3) lowering the interest rate paid by loan recipients from the going federal rate (which averaged 4.25 percent in 1965-66 and 5.375 percent in 1969) to a uniform rate of 3 percent per year on the unpaid balance; and (4) expanding the partial "forgiveness" clause at the rate of 10 percent per year for a maximum of five years of full-time employment as a professional nurse by allowing up to 100 percent cancellation, at the rate of 15 percent annually for full-time hospital employment in an area designated as having a substantial shortage of nurses.

The HMA also established a new scholarship program which, in effect, constituted an expansion of the program added to the NTA in 1966. Specifically: (1) grants were authorized to eligible individual nursing schools for scholarship programs; (2) the matching funds requirement was dropped; (3) the annual amount to be awarded to eligible schools was set at $2,000 times one-tenth of the school's full-time enrollment; (4) each school was permitted to award grants on the basis of a student's needs and resources up to a maximum $1,500 per year; and (5) a school was permitted to transfer up to 20 percent of the amount of federal funds received for its loan program to its scholarship program, or vice versa.

All other provisions of Title II of the HMA involved relatively minor changes in the program established by the NTA. Principal among these were modifications in the Construction Grants section which: (1) authorized the Secretary of HEW to increase the maximum federal share of school construction costs from one-half to two-thirds in cases where he determined that "unusual circumstances" prevailed; (2) allowed collegiate programs to include areas needed for continuing education (nondegree) programs as eligible space in applying for construction grants; and (3) eliminated separate appropriations for collegiate and diploma or associate degree schools of nursing.

Table 2 summarizes experience under the HMA in terms of appropriations and awards relative to authorizations. Although considerably fewer funds were actually appropriated than were authorized, it is apparent that there were no longer insufficient eligible applicants to award most of the appropriated funds to in major program areas.

The Nurse Training Act of 1971 expanded Title II of the HMA through fiscal 1974. Specifically, it authorized: $120 million for construction grants; $83 million for special project grants; $248 million for institutional grants (which were separated from the special project grants authorization); $7 million for a new program of interest subsidies and loan guarantees on nonfederal construction loans (with the stipulations that these subsidies be limited to an amount sufficient to reduce the interest rate on construction loans by no more than 3 percent per year and that the guarantees not bring the federal share of construction costs to more than 90 percent); $30 million for grants to schools that are in serious financial distress because of a need to maintain the quality of their programs or to meet accreditation requirements; $24 million for start-up grants with a maximum of $100,000 per fiscal year, to plan, develop, and initiate new nurse-training programs; $66 million for the professional Nurse Traineeship program; $90.5 million (plus the amount necessary to fulfill previous commitments through 1977) for student loans; $172.5 million for the scholarship grants program (based upon the allocation formula in the

Table 2
Authorization, Appropriations, and Awards under the Provisions
of Title II of the Health Manpower Act, 1968
(in Thousands of Dollars)

Provision	Fiscal 1970			Fiscal 1971			Total		
	Authorized	Appropriated	Awarded	Authorized	Appropriated	Awarded	Authorized	Appropriated	Awarded
Construction	25,000	8,000	11,414	35,000	9,500	8,232	60,000	17,500	19,646
Special project	15,000*	8,400	7,000	15,000*	11,500	11,350	30,000	19,900	18,350
Institutional grants	20,000*	0	0	25,000*	0	0	45,000	0	0
Student loans	20,000	16,360	12,281	21,000	17,110	16,752	41,000	33,470	29,033
Traineeships	15,000	10,470	10,468	19,000	10,470	10,470	34,000	20,940	20,938
Scholarships	32,000†	7,200	10,727	33,000†	17,000	17,000	65,000	24,200	27,727
Total	127,000	50,430	51,890	148,000	65,580	63,804	275,000	116,010	115,694

*Section 808 authorized $35,000,000 in FY 1970 and $40,000,000 in FY 1971 for the sum of Special Projects grants, plus Institutional grants, with the added provision that the first $15,000,000 appropriated in each year be for Special Projects.
†Scholarship authorizations were computed from the formula provided in section 860 (b) of HMA.

act and HEW enrollment projections), plus an undetermined amount to allow students who receive scholarships before 1 July 1974 to continue or complete their training; and $15 million for grants and contracts to identify and assist potential nursing students and to publicize sources of financial aid.

The NTA of 1971 also contained several new provisions—namely, it:

Prohibited discrimination by participating schools on the basis of sex.

Liberalized the construction grants program by increasing the maximum federal share to 75 percent for major remodeling needed to increase enrollment or for new facilities which will provide a major expansion of teaching activities (or in "unusual circumstances") and 67 percent for all other construction projects.

Enlarged the list of special projects eligible for assistance to include mergers and cooperation between training facilities, development of interdisciplinary training programs, relating advances in other fields to nursing, increasing opportunities for disadvantaged students, and the provision of retraining for inactive nurses.

Established a new formula for computing a school's annual entitlement under the institutional grant program.

Increased the maximum size of student loans to $2,500 per year, and $10,000 in total, with up to 85 percent "forgiveness" for full-time employment in any public or nonprofit facility for five years (15 percent for the first three years, and 20 percent for the last two).

Raised the maximum annual scholarship to $2,000. Half-time students were made eligible for the program, and participating schools were entitled to receive an amount equal to $3,000 times one-tenth of the number of full-time students enrolled to finance the program.

Assessment of Impact

As of this date, appropriation figures and partial awards data are available only for 1972. It will probably be at least another year before the final figures on appropriations and awards are known. Nevertheless, sufficient data are now available to assess the impact of the Nurse Training Act of 1964 and, at least partially, that of its subsequent extensions and revisions. At the time the Nurse Training Act was established, it was announced that this would be a five-year effort to achieve what the Surgeon General's Consulting Group on Nursing (SGCGN) had set as a feasible goal for 1970: "To increase the supply of professional nurses in practice to about 680,000." The framers of the Act accepted the SGCGN's contention that, "to meet this goal, schools of nursing must produce 53,000 graduates a year by 1969—a 75 percent increase over 1961." The basic goal of 680,000 active nurses by 1970 was actually achieved a year ahead of schedule (1969). Viewed in this light, it would appear the NTA was eminently successful. However, this goal would not have been obtained—even by 1970—if it had really depended upon producing "53,000 nursing school graduates by 1969." The actual number of graduates in 1969 was 42,196. This figure is only slightly higher than the 41,000 projected graduations for 1969 made by the SGCGN, assuming that "nursing schools would continue to draw the present proportion of girls in the age group finishing high school." Thus, the actual increase in 1969 graduations was only 10 percent of the increase which the SGCGN said would be necessary to attain the nurse employment level achieved in 1969.

These figures raise two interesting and important questions. First, what factors made it possible to achieve the SGCGN's nurse employment goal a year in advance even though graduations were only slightly higher than the level projected for them in the absence of the NTA? Second, why was the impact of the NTA so much smaller in terms of increased graduations than the SGCGN had anticipated?

We do not know the full answer to the first question at this time. However, Robert T. Deane and I recently developed an econometric model of the nurse market which is capable of providing some of the answers.[2] Preliminary results attribute the 1969 employment level to increased nurse participation rates, and to the movement of the abnormally large 1946-48 graduating classes from low to high labor force participation age cohorts. The higher participation rates were, in turn, due to unusually large nurse salary increases associated with the advent of Medicare and Medicaid. Increases in graduations had almost no effect on the growth of total nurse employment. Furthermore, as the close conformity of the 1969 actual graduations to the SGCGN's projections for the present trend implies, most of the increase in graduations is attributable to the growth in the number of female high school graduates. The remainder is probably explained by the observed increase in nurse salaries.

With respect to the second question posed, why NTA's impact was less

2. Robert T. Deane and Donald E. Yett, "Nurse Market Policy Simulations Using an Econometric Model" (paper presented at the 48th Annual Conference of the Western Economic Association, Claremont, California, 17 Aug. 1973).

than SGCGN anticipated, there are two ways in which the Nurse Training Act might have been able to increase the annual number of graduations. First, by providing financial support to needy students the NTA might have made it possible for some to remain in school who otherwise would have dropped out. Second, the Act's provisions might have induced some individuals to attend nursing school who otherwise would have chosen a different career—i.e., marginal entrants. The evidence is clear on both scores. Between 1963 and 1968, the nursing school dropout rate fluctuated, with no discernable trend, around its long-term value of one-third. Likewise, it has been estimated that the *maximum* number of marginal entrants attributable to the Act was extremely small. The *maximum* number of marginal students who enrolled in nursing schools as a result of the Act can be computed using data in the 1970 report of the secretary of HEW on the NTA. In this report it is assumed that *any* difference in admissions to nursing school between the projected trend and the actual amount can be attributed to the effects of the Act. On the basis of this assumption, the total number of marginal entrants due to the NTA program was reported to be 3,990 for the entire 1965-67 period. Using the average dropout rate for this period (33 percent), these figures implied that the increase in enrollment of marginal entrants resulted in approximately 2,660 graduates over the years 1968 to 1970.

These simple calculations illustrate, of course, the difficulties encountered in general by programs designed to increase employment via training subsidies. That is, in order to maximize the benefit of such programs, it is essential that the funds be allocated to prospective students who otherwise would *not* have enrolled in the training program (marginal entrants) or who, by the same token, would *not* have completed their training (dropouts). In nursing, as well as in other professions, it is extremely difficult to identify who these individuals are exactly. Consequently, it is not practical to limit financial support (e.g., forgivable loans and, later in the program, scholarships) to marginal entrants. This means the support provided to all recipients must be sufficient to afford a positive financial reward for a career in nursing relative to alternative careers. Otherwise, little if any support will go to the marginal entrants.

If all of the other advantages and disadvantages of alternative careers were equal, we would expect a person to choose the one with the highest present value of future earnings relative to the costs of required training. In this context, marginal entrants are those for whom the costs of training and the expected earnings are the deciding factors in selecting a particular career. These two factors can be combined by calculating the internal rate of return associated with an investment in one type of training (e.g., a diploma, A.A., or B.A. degree in nursing), which can then be compared with the returns on other types of training (e.g., general B.A. or B.S. degree) or with the returns on alternative investment opportunities (e.g., stocks and bonds). There are technical reasons for preferring to compare present values, or rates of return over cost, of alternative investment options (including career choices). Nevertheless, many economists continue to employ the internal-rate-of-return approach, because experience has shown that the alternative methods generally lead to the same conclusions, and the rate-of-return approach has considerable intuitive appeal.

Internal rate of return on training

With this in mind, I would now like to review with you some calculations of the rate of return on investments in nurse training relative to the rates for alternative types of training. I will then demonstrate how the rates of return for nurses were affected by the loan (and subsequent scholarship) provisions of the NTA.

The internal rate of return for investment option i is the value of r which satisfies the equality:

$$\int_{O}^{T} [R_i(t) - O_i(t) - C_i(t)]e^{-rt}dt = O,$$

where

$R_i(t)$ = the receipts stream;

$O_i(t)$ = the opportunity cost stream;

$C_i(t)$ = the direct cost stream; and

t = the unit of time.

A great many nonwage factors should be considered as part of the returns stream for any given investment in training. Most of these factors are extremely difficult, if not impossible, to include in making actual estimates. However, minimum estimates can be made on the basis of net earnings. These estimates assume that the investment in training must be at least equal to the resulting net increase in the individual's productivity (i.e., earning power). Table 3 presents such estimates of the internal rates of return on various amounts of investment in training for nurses and for females in general. They are based on year-round average earnings data (including those received for part-time work during the training period). The opportunity cost streams were taken to be the year-round earnings for the next lower (i.e., immediately preceeding) educational level. The earnings and cost streams were survivor-weighted, and appropriate tax rates were applied to the earnings streams.

Table 3

Internal Rates of Return for All Females with Post-High School Education and for Nurses Based on Year-Round 1966 Earnings (in Percentage)

Category of Worker (By Level of Post-High School Education)*	Potential Earnings (Continuous Employment, 100% Participation)			Expected Earnings — Predetermined Participation Pattern: Average Rate for Females with 1-3 Years College			Expected Earnings — Predetermined Participation Pattern: Average Rate for Females with 4 Years College			Expected Earnings — Varying Participation Pattern (Average Rate for Specific Occupation and Educational Level)		
	No NTA Support	Loan‖	With Scholarship◆	No NTA Support	Loan‖	With Scholarship◆	No NTA Support	Loan‖	With Scholarship◆	No NTA Support	Loan‖	With Scholarship◆
All Females												
1-3 years college	5.1	...	...	1.6	...	...	2.4	...	...	2.4	...	...
4 years college	6.7	...	...	2.7	...	...	3.5	...	...	10.0	...	...
5 or more years college	4.0	...	...	...	...	...	...	...	...	7.9	...	...
Nurses												
2 years of training†	13.1	14.2	16.6	6.9	...	9.4	8.4	...	10.3	17.4	64.3	26.7
3 years of training:												
Without maintenance provided	8.3	8.9	10.3	3.9	...	5.1	4.8	...	5.8	11.8	32.3	17.6
With maintenance only	9.3	10.0	12.1	4.6	...	6.1	5.6	...	6.8	14.1	42.4	24.8
With average maintenance only‡	8.4	9.0	10.6	4.0	...	5.2	4.9	...	5.9	12.0	33.3	18.2
With average maintenance and part-time earnings‡	9.1	9.9	11.9	4.5	...	6.0	5.5	...	6.6	13.8	41.0	23.7
With maintenance and part-time earnings	10.2	11.1	13.8	5.2	...	7.0	6.3	...	7.7	16.8	55.1	39.9
4 years of training	7.3	8.0	9.2	3.1	...	4.3	3.9	...	4.9	9.8	21.9	14.0
5 or more years of training§	3.9	4.3	...	...	...	...	...	...	3.4**	4.2	10.1	...

Note: All figures shown are survivor-adjusted, after tax, and inclusive of student earnings, except those nurse figures marked "maintenance only." Participation rates are applied up to age 80, except that in the case of potential earnings 100 percent participation rates are applied up to age 65.

*Persons with 1 to 3 years of college were assumed to be in training an average of 2 years, and persons with 5 or more years of college were assumed to be in training for 6 years. Beginning with the fifth year of training, opportunity cost for those with 5 or more years training was assumed to be the average earnings for persons with 4 years of training in the same age-occupation cohort.

†Nurses with 2 years of training were given the same earnings streams after graduation as those with 3 years.

‡Average maintenance was 50 percent in 1966.

§The opportunity cost for the first four years of the 6-year program is the gross earnings of female high school graduates and for the remaining years is the gross earnings of females with baccalaureate degrees.

‖The loans are assumed to be received each year of training and full payment is made by paying back one-tenth of the total amount loaned in each of the first five working years. The actual average sizes of the loans in fiscal 1966 were: 2-year programs, $686; 3-year programs, $541; 4-year programs, $652; and 6-year programs, $630.

◆Assuming $1,000 scholarship per year during training in diploma, associate, and baccalaureate degree nursing programs.

**Labor force participation rates of females with 5 or more years college were used for this figure.

Two sets of calculations were made to examine the relative attractiveness of nursing under alternative assumptions regarding the appropriate labor-force participation patterns to be considered. Specifically, estimates were made assuming that:

1. A woman's labor-force participation pattern is largely predetermined before her career choice is made and thus, is independent of the occupation and associated educational level selected.

2. The expected participation pattern varies (as do earnings, training costs, and length of training) with a woman's occupational choice.

Since the number of possible predetermined patterns appropriate for the first set of calculations is virtually infinite, the following were selected as useful examples: (1) continuous employment from graduation to retirement at age 65; (2) the average labor-force participation pattern for women with 1-3 years of post-high school education; and (3) the average pattern for all female college graduates. (In the last two cases the individual was presumed to be "professionally dead" at age 80.) The first of these patterns assumes a 100 percent participation rate for a female employee and so yields the maximum (potential) earnings. The other two assumed patterns take a more realistic view of female participation rates based on averages for female employees in all occupations and therefore yield lower (expected) earnings.

For the second set of calculations the average participation rate for each occupation and/or level of education was employed. Thus, in this sense, the expected earnings differential for a nurse age 25 would be the average earnings for nurses at that age times their average labor-force participation rate minus the average earnings of female high school graduates of the same age times the latter's labor-force participation rate.

As shown in Table 3, even without NTA loan or scholarship assistance, all forms of nurse training compared favorably with investments in the same number of years of college education.[3] The observed difference in the rate of return on a baccalaureate degree in nursing and a general B.A. were too small to be significant. However, the much greater differentials in the returns on both two- and three-year nurse-training programs and general A.A. or B.A. degrees deserves closer attention. In the case of the three-year diploma programs the higher returns were probably not suf-

---

3. The only exception being "5 or more years of training," where the two options were about equal when the same participation rates were applied to both the earnings streams and to the opportunity cost streams.

ficient to offset their nonfinancial disadvantages—e.g., apprenticeship type work requirements, restrictions on social life, little or no access to job opportunities other than in nursing, etc.—and the steady decline in number of applicants was seen as a factor contributing to the substantial reduction in the number of such programs. Other factors often mentioned as bearing on this reduction include: the NLN accreditation program; the ANA endorsement of a nurse hierarchy which would greatly limit promotional opportunities for diploma graduates in comparison to those with B.A.'s and worsening cost/benefit ratios associated with such programs from the point of view of the hospitals which have traditionally operated them.

The large differential in favor of A.A. nursing programs relative to the same or larger amounts of general college training may be partially explainable in terms of data pecularities. First, a large percentage of the females with 1-3 years of college are dropouts rather than general A.A. degree holders. Thus, they would not be expected to earn much more than female high school graduates. Second, nurses with A.A. degrees may not be as well paid as diploma graduates. And, since separate figures were not available, the necessary assumption of equal pay may have resulted in an upward bias in the A.A. nurse earnings figures. Nevertheless, it is almost inconceivable that the entire differential can be explained in terms of inadequate statistics. Thus, it would have been safe to predict a substantial growth in A.A. nursing programs—with or without NTA support.

Table 3 also shows the effects of the partially forgivable NTA student loans and scholarships on the returns to investments in nurse training. The student loan calculations were based on that section of the Act which provided for a maximum loan amount of $1000 with 10 percent forgiveness for each year employed in nursing up to a maximum of five years. As noted earlier, subsequent changes in the legislation have increased the maximum loan amount (to $2,500) and the size of the forgiveness (to 85 percent). Given these changes, and the relative rise in nurse earnings since 1966, the figures presented represent minimum estimates of the loan program's impact on the returns to investments in nurse training. In all cases—except those involving expected participation rates specific to different occupations and levels of education—they show a consistent but small (seldom more than one percentage point) increase in the differential favoring nursing training over general higher education. Moreover, the relative rankings among the basic nurse training programs remained the same.

The only calculations which were greatly affected by the introduction of the NTA loan program were those involving expected participation rates specific to different occupations and levels of education. Before the student loan figures were incorporated into these calculations, both baccalaureate and post graduate nurse training exhibited slightly lower rates of return than did the comparable classifications for all females with college education. However, the introduction of student loans brought about such dramatic increases in their rates of return that all nurse training programs became preferred over the same level of college training for all females. Indeed, these rates of return were, in most cases, doubled or even tripled. These results indicate that the only marginal entrants who would be strongly influenced by the NTA loan program are those who would be willing to work all of the first five years after graduation to take maximum advantage of the forgiveness provision (but would otherwise follow the participation pattern typical of nonnurses with specified levels of education). Undoubtedly such individuals found the NTA loans extremely attractive. However, there were too few of them to assure the success of the program. By 30 June 1966 requests had been received to de-obligate $2.6 million of federal funds awarded under the loan program; and in 1967 only about 75 percent of the funds appropriated for loans were awarded.

Apparently the poor results obtained in the initial years of the NTA loan program were due to a lack of demand for such loans rather than to insufficient appropriations. Subsequent increases in the earnings of nurses and more liberal loan provisions may result in an increased demand. However, this cannot yet be determined, owing to the fact that recent spending limitations have restricted total awards to levels below those in previous years. If, in the future, there is sufficient demand to warrant larger NTA loan appropriations—and there is also a significant rise in the proportion of nursing school applicants to female high school graduates—this would imply that the loans were attracting more marginal entrants into nursing. It would not, however, imply a decline in the number of nonmarginal students who would also be receiving such support. Accordingly, the total amount of support necessary to *add* an additional student would continue to exceed the size of the now liberalized average loan by a considerable amount.

Since scholarships, by definition, do not require repayment, they reduce the cost of training, and thereby increase its rate of return, without at the same time saddling the recipient with a long-term obligation. Thus, possessing the advantages but not the disadvantages of student loans, scholarships should be a more effective device for attracting marginal nursing school entrants—provided, of course, they do not go primarily to students who would have enrolled without such aid.

As has been explained, the NTA was amended in 1966 to include a scholarship program. Initially, the maximum a nursing school could award was $1,000.[4] Moreover, in an effort to direct these funds toward marginal students, the legislation specified that they were given only to students of exceptional financial need who otherwise would be unable to enter or remain in school. Subsequent legislation increased the maximum annual scholarship to $1,500 in 1968, and $2,000 in 1971. However—as in the case of the loan program—the estimates of the impact of these scholarships on the expected returns on nurse training are based on 1966 earnings, and assume the maximum 1966 annual scholarships, so that the effect on current returns to nurse training are understated.

The figures given in Table 3 indicate that the maximum nursing school scholarships raised the potential return (i.e., assuming 100 percent participation to age 65) by only about two to four percentage points. However, these increases were, nonetheless, almost double those of the maximum NTA loan. Like the NTA student loans, the scholarships had virtually no effect on the relation of the rates of return of the different types of nurse-training programs.

Except on a potential return basis, direct comparisons of the estimated impacts of the NTA loan and scholarship provisions may be misleading for several reasons. First, data on the actual average size of the scholarships in 1966 were not available. Thus, the comparisons made are in terms of the maximum possible scholarships and actual average loans. Second—and most important—the estimate of the impact of the loan program was based on the assumption that the recipient took full advantage of the forgiveness feature then in effect. *All* of the loan impact calculations reported in Table 3 assume 100 percent labor force participation for five years after graduation.

Despite the upward bias in the loan estimates relative to the scholarship estimates,[5] the latter were higher than the former on the basis of earnings streams as weighted by the rate of participation of female college graduates. When the participation rates for females with one to three years

---

4. Matching funds were authorized for grants to nursing schools so that they could award scholarships to qualified needy students in the amount of $800, or one-half of the total financial aid that such a student receives from other sources of scholarship funds up to that amount. An additional $200 was awarded to scholarship recipients who finished the preceding year in the upper half of their classes. Thus, it was possible to receive a maximum award of $1,000 annually under this program.

5. The increase in the net earnings streams caused by the assumption of 100 percent labor force participation in the first five years after graduation from nursing school may more than offset the decrease in the net earnings streams caused by assuming that 50 percent of the loan was paid back. Thus, in some cases, the returns from an NTA loan were estimated to be greater than those from a scholarship of the same dollar amount.

of college were employed, the maximum scholarships yielded rates which were only about the same as those based upon average NTA loans. Only with respect to the occupation- and education-specific rates of return were there substantial differences in the estimates. Any marginal entrant who is willing to adjust her labor force participation rate as a *consequence* of her career choice (rather than the reverse) will find both the loans and the scholarships attractive; but, if she also seeks to take maximum advantage of the foregiveness feature, she will find the former more attractive than the latter. Indeed, in the case of such an individual, the greatest impact would be achieved by offering her 100 percent forgiveness spread out over a longer period of time.

On the basis of the foregoing analysis, it is not surprising that the evidence indicates that the scholarships were more sought after than the loans. After a slow start in 1967, practically all of the funds appropriated for scholarships were awarded in 1968, and all those appropriated in 1969 were awarded. This is in direct contrast with experience during the earlier years of the loan program when some federal funds had to be de-obligated, and subsequent appropriations were cut to bring them into line with actual awards.[6]

The apparent success of the scholarship program was a predictable consequence of its raising the expected return on nurse training without requiring a long-term obligation on the part of the recipient. Indeed, in view of recent steps to liberalize the program, its further so-called success would seem to be assured—at least in these terms. On the other hand, it is virtually impossible to judge whether the scholarship program has been successful in terms of its avowed goal of providing support to students who otherwise would be unable to enter or remain in nursing schools. It is known that the proportion of nursing students who drop out for financial reasons is very small. Thus, the goal of the scholarship program could only be achieved by bringing marginal entrants into nursing schools. To the extent that scholarships have gone to nonmarginal entrants, they have replaced other sources of assistance to financially needy students who, nonetheless, would still have attended nursing schools.

6. In fiscal 1965 $3,100,000 were appropriated for the establishment of student loan funds, of which $1,608,000 were remaining in established funds at the end of the year. Schools were encouraged to retain these funds as a carry-over for the next year's operation of their loan programs. In fiscal 1966 $8,900,000 were appropriated for this program. These funds were sufficient to cover the entire amounts requested by eligible schools. Indeed, by 30 June 1966 requests had been received to de-obligate $2,600,000 of federal funds awarded under the program. In fiscal 1967 $16,900,000 were appropriated, but only $12,677,000 were awarded. The Division of Nursing (UPHS) speculated that the 1966 ammendment which authorized revolving loan funds would make possible the use of this carry-over.

There is no reliable way to determine whether a particular needy student would or would not have entered nurse training without a scholarship. If future studies indicate a rise in the proportion of students coming from low-income families, this would be indirect evidence that the goal was, indeed, being accomplished. Less conclusive evidence of some possible recent success is provided by figures which show a sizable increase in the number of associate-degree students receiving NTA scholarships. The shorter length of these training programs makes them more attractive to needy students, and, therefore, the probability that scholarships actually go to marginal entrants is higher in the case of associate degree programs.

Experience with other provisions of NTA

Construction. Experience to date with respect to the construction, special project, and the institutional grant provisions of the NTA can be summarized briefly. Concerning construction, it should be pointed out that from the beginning of the NTA, virtually all of the funds appropriated for construction grants to baccalaurate programs were actually awarded. However, only about 60 percent of the funds appropriated for diploma and associate degree programs were awarded in 1966, and none of the funds appropriated for these programs were awarded in 1967. The 1966 amendment which permitted transfer of unused funds between types of program largely eliminated this situation.

In 1966-67, less than 20 percent of the construction grant funds went for building characterized as being for new "first-year places" as opposed to that for "student places maintained." By 1968-69, the proportion had increased to 50 percent. This change was due primarily to the rapid growth of associate degree programs, where 85 percent of the funds were used to create new first-year positions. However, these newly created positions served mainly to replace the large numbers of diploma places which were not being maintained. The total net increase in first positions, therefore, was small—which is not surprising given that 1963 nursing school capacity was already adequate for the expected 1966 enrollment on the basis of existing trends. Unless the liberalized loan and scholarship programs draw considerably more marginal entrants into nursing, it is reasonable to expect that the *net* increase in first-year positions will continue to be small—with the bulk of the funds being used to maintain existing places, or to replace existing places not being maintained (primarily because of the closing of diploma schools) with new positions in associate degree and baccalaurate programs.

Special projects and institutional grants. The special project grants program established by the NTA has been quite successful. Virtually all of the funds appropriated by Congress for such grants have been awarded. The initial 1964 NTA grants to enable nursing schools to expand and strengthen their teaching programs reportedly benefited over 49,000 students in 332 nursing programs. On the basis of this experience—and of the fact that these projects involve little or no additional cost to the school—it would be reasonable to expect this to be one of the most successful provisions of the nurse-training legislation. Moreover, when the scope and eligibility of this program were broadened it was necessary in 1968 for Congress to set priorities to guide the allocation of funds available for such grants.

One of the less successful provisions of the NTA involved payments to diploma schools to help defray the costs of additional enrollments expected as a result of the Act. Specifically, any accredited nonprofit diploma school was entitled to receive $250 for each student who had an NTA loan and also for each student in excess of its average full-time enrollment during the period from fiscal 1962 through fiscal 1964 (up to a maximum of $100 times its full-time enrollment).

Shortly after the NTA was enacted, it was estimated that

> including both the value of her clinical services and the [$250] federal subsidy, the marginal return from an additional [diploma school] student is $850. Thus, only hospital schools [near the lowest end of the $750 to $1,500 range of estimated average outlays on room and board alone] would be willing to accept an additional student under these conditions. Moreover, no school which has reached the ceiling, where its subsidy for an additional student is only $100 per year, would be willing to accept another student solely on the basis of this subsidy. If the school must increase its enrollment, however, in order to fully utilize its [NTA] loan fund, the marginal return from an additional student would be $1,100 rather than $850. Under these conditions a school would be willing to increase its enrollment, unless its room and board costs were near the maximum of the estimated range or unless it would have to expand its staff or facilities in order to accept additional students.[7]

Under these circumstances, it is not surprising that less than half of the $6,500,000 appropriated for payments to diploma schools were actually awarded in fiscal years 1965 and 1966, or that only 20 percent of the funds awarded were based upon straight increases in enrollment. Also, it should be noted that 30 percent of the payments were based solely on the number of students participating in the NTA loan program, and that 50 percent were based upon a combination of the loan recipient factor with one or more of the other components of the formula. It was reasonable to expect that the 1966 amendment permitting schools to set up NTA loan programs

---

7. Donald E. Yett, "The Nursing Shortage and the Nurse Training Act of 1964," *Industrial and Labor Relations Review* 19 (Jan. 1966): 195.

on a revolving fund basis—without the necessity of securing matching funds—would at least lead to an increase in the former percentage and, possibly, the latter as well. Indeed, after the amendment approximately 40 percent of the payments to diploma schools were awarded solely on the basis of number of NTA loan recipients, while the proportion based upon a combination of factors including loan recipients remained virtually constant. Nevertheless, this was not sufficient to close the gap between appropriations and awards. Appropriations were cut back from $6,000,000 in 1967 to $3,000,000 in 1968 and 1969, all of which were awarded.

Title II of the Health Manpower Act of 1968 extended institutional grant eligibility to associate degree and baccalaureate, as well as diploma, schools of nursing. In addition, the formula for calculating a school's entitlement was liberalized. The HMA also specified, however, that the first $15 million of an appropriation for special-projects and institutional grants had to be allocated for special projects; and, since only $8,400,000 and $11,500,000 were appropriated in fiscal 1970 and 1971, respectively, no institutional grants were awarded under the HMA.

The Nurse Training Act of 1971 authorized separate appropriations for special project and institutional grants. It also established a new formula involving a major change of emphasis. The original formula had implied that nursing schools would be unwilling to accept sizable increases in enrollment without operating subsidies. In effect, its authors assumed that the loan program would bring forth a larger number of applicants than nursing schools would accept without additional support. However, experience amply demonstrates that the anticipated surge of nursing school applicants did not materialize and that nursing school admission policies, therefore, were not a major bottleneck preventing the implementation of what otherwise would have been a successful student recruiting program. The new formula implicitly recognizes that, under present circumstances, nursing schools may not be able to exert effective action to increase the total number of admissions. Consequently, while maintaining basic program support, it offers a sizable incentive for them to take action in one area where they should be able to exert control—namely, lowering student attrition rates.

Specifically, the new institutional grant formula combines a $100 payment to the school for each increase in first-year enrollments, and $250 general support for each continuing student enrolled, with $500 for each student who graduates that year ($900 if the student graduates from a nurse-midwife program). Thus, each increase in first-year enrollment brings the school an additional $350 the first year, and $250 annually until the year of the enrollee's graduation, at which time the school receives a $500 payment. Under the circumstances, if adequate funds are appropriated (and awarded), the new institutional grant program could represent a successful effort to stimulate an increase in the number of *graduate* nurses—even if admissions remain little affected by the overall program.

Nurse Traineeship Program. Another important provision of the NTA and subsequent nurse-training legislation was the continuation of the Nurse Traineeship Program initiated in 1956. Under this program funds are made available to support short-term and long-term training for graduate nurses in the areas of administration, supervision, teaching, and nurse specialties. The short-term courses are generally workshops for development or improvement of skills. Long-term traineeships, on the other hand, typically cover additional formal education beyond the basic RN level. That is, they provide associate degree and diploma graduates with support in completing the requirements for a baccalaureate degree and graduates of the latter program with support for postbaccalaureate studies.

Although Table 3 indicates that the returns on postgraduate nurse training are much lower than for basic programs, it should be emphasized that this calculation is based on a comparison with rates for a recent female high-school graduate. The *marginal* rate of return on post graduate work to an RN with a baccalaureate degree is the appropriate measure to apply in evaluating this aspect of the Traineeship Program. Calculations parallel to those in Table 3 were made of the rate of return on *additional* nurse training beyond graduation from baccalaureate programs, and on the rates of return to associate degree and diploma graduates who go on to obtain baccalaureate degrees in nursing. These figures, based on 1966 data, were estimated on the assumption that an associate degree or diploma RN can complete her work for the baccalaureate in two years. In the first year she receives an average of $4,080 to cover expenses; and in the second year she receives no support. Training cost for each of the two additional years is $791 per year. Her forgone earnings in all years are the salary she would have received as a practicing 1-3 years graduate nurse. Similarly, a postgraduate nursing student was assumed to receive an average of $5,464 for each of two years' additional study. Her forgone earnings are, of course, the salary she would have received as a 4-year graduate nurse; and, again, the direct costs of training are $791 per year. The resulting estimates indicated potential rates of return (i.e., assuming 100 percent participation to age 65) of 8.7 and 8.8 percent, respectively, on the additional training for an associate degree and a diploma school graduate to obtain a baccalaureate nursing degree. And, in both cases, the rate of return on an occupation- and education-specific basis was estimated to be 4.2 percent. These figures raise doubt that Nurse Traineeship will entice very many associate degree and diploma school graduates to go on for baccalaureate degrees.[8]

By contrast, the rate of return on postgraduate training to a baccalaureate nursing degree holder was estimated to be in excess of 80 percent on either a potential or occupation- and education-specific basis. Clearly, the Nurse Traineeship Program provides a strong incentive for RNs to seek additional education beyond a baccalaureate degree in nursing. Essentially, it offers them the opportunity to acquire the education necessary to compete for the highest-paid positions in nursing, without, at the same time, requiring a substantial financial sacrifice during the period of additional training. In view of these results it is not surprising that the Nurse Traineeship Program has had a history of notable success.[9] On the other hand, in view of the low returns on further basic training for associate degree and diploma graduates, it is doubtful that this aspect of the program would have much attraction except as an entree to postgraduate work. Finally, the magnitude of the rates of return on postgraduate work make it safe to predict that the funds allotted for this program will continue to be chronically oversubscribed[10] and most of the funds will be used to support graduate students.

In conclusion, it should be pointed out that reports by nursing and public health experts indicate they believe the so-called shortage of nurses is a less serious problem now than it was a decade—or even half a decade—ago. In 1963 the SGCGN predicted that if the then-present trend continued there would be only 41,000 nurses graduated in 1969, and that the number of professional nurses in practice would be 200,000 less than the number needed by January 1970. Moreover the group maintained that, even if what it saw as the feasible goal of 53,000 graduates by 1969 were achieved via a massive program of federal support for nurse training, there would be a shortage of 170,000 nurses relative to the number needed.

Considering that the actual number of nurses graduated in 1969 was only 42,196, despite the fact that most of the recommendations of the SGCGN were enacted, a shortage close to the 200,000 figure would not, therefore, have been surprising. However, in 1969 the U.S. Public Health Service (Division of Nursing) estimated the number of employed

---

8. About 2,200 diploma and associate degree graduates obtained baccalaureate nursing degrees in 1968. This compares with about 2,500 in 1962.

9. Between fiscal 1957 and 1969, an estimated 25,161 RNs received long-term traineeships. Of these, 14,286 were for post-baccalaureate and 632 for post-master's study. Also, between fiscal 1960 and 1969, it is estimated that 37,991 nurses attended a total of 1,079 short-term training courses.

10. In fiscal 1970 only 74 percent of the Nurse Traineeship requests could be funded.

registered nurses was 170,000 less than the 1970 need. Then in 1971, for the first time in over 20 years, there was a decline in the estimated shortage of nurses. Specifically, the deficit between supply and need was placed at 157,000.

Moreover, the period 1966 to 1969 witnessed a dramatic increase in all measures of nurse remuneration relative to any reasonable reference group. Some might interpret this relative wage increase as further evidence of a shortage of nurses. However, I am inclined to believe it indicated that a correction of the shortage had begun to gather momentum. This interpretation is, moreover, consistent with reports of a substantial decline in job vacancies for hospital nurses. If it is true that the nurse market has been experiencing a correction in response to a chronic shortage, one might well wonder what finally caused the process to get underway.

Correction of the Market for Nurses

In regard to correction of the market for nurses, the establishment of the Medicare-Medicaid program in the mid-1960s had two important effects. First, it increased the demand for nurses; and, second, it reduced the elasticity of the demand curve. According to at least one contemporary report, the first of these effects was not particularly large. The U.S. Public Health Service estimated that the need for nurses increased by only about 5 percent as a result of this legislation. On the other hand, the reduction in the elasticity of demand may have been considerable, as yet another opportunity was given to hospital administrators to pass on cost increases to third parties without any resulting decrease in services demanded. As one expert explained, "the cost-pass-through provisions of the insurance mechanisms and Medicare-Medicaid are providing the financial support for unilateral efforts by hospitals to improve salaries, personnel policies, job content, and managerial methods."[11]

In addition, there are indications that demand was nearing the upper limit of the discontinuous portion of the marginal factor cost curve for nurses faced by oligopsonistic hopsital employers. Combined with the other forces pushing up demands, the Medicare-Medicaid increase may have been sufficient to push the demand curve out of the discontinuous range, thereby precipitating a series of wage adjustments toward new higher equilibrium levels in the affected markets. At the same time, many hospitals apparently sought to avoid collective bargaining by nurses by

11. Ronald L. Miller, "Development and Structure of Collective Bargaining among Nurses: Part II," *Personnel Journal* 50 (Mar. 1971): 225.

voluntarily adopting higher salary scales patterned after several widely publicized negotiated agreements.

In any event, nurse salaries rose by double the rate of all relevant reference groups between the years 1966 and 1969. Despite the low elasticity of nurse supply, such large salary increases, combined with the changing age structure of the stock of nurses, gave rise to a sizeable increase in the nurse labor force participation rate. The higher nurse labor force participation rate, in turn, contributed to a substantial rise in nurse employment. Hospital nurse vacancies declined from their all-time high in the early 1960s to levels which were at or below those of the immediate post war years.[12] The important point to bear in mind is that these improvements were due almost exclusively to demographic and market forces.

Although thus far, at least, the number of additional new graduates attributable to federal support for nurse training has been too small to affect the nurse market one way or the other, the federal program has been expanded and liberalized step by step, to the point where there is a strong possibility that it will have large future impact. Maximum loans under the NTA are now two and one-half times their original size, with lower interest rates and forgiveness of up to 85 percent in five years. Maximum scholarship awards are now double the original amount established in 1966. Moreover, nursing schools can now participate in both programs without the necessity of securing matching funds. Indeed, any nursing school which does not participate to the maximum extent its circumstances will allow stands to lose considerable benefits in terms of lower institutional grant awards. Granted that the program is all carrot and no stick, the carrot has grown, at least potentially, to an unusually large size. If enough of the authorized funds are appropriated and awarded, a school which is hard-pressed financially can now be kept going via the enlarged special project grants provision. Likewise, if authorized funds for construction grants are eventually awarded, a school with a physical plant in need of renovation and/or expansion could get up to 90 percent of the costs of these improvements from federal funds. Deficient faculty can be upgraded via the Nurse Traineeship Program. Finally, for schools which meet the eligibility requirements, each increase in enrollment brings a $100 bonus, over and above its annual $250 per student operating subsidy, and another bonus of $250 when the student graduates. Predictably, attrition

---

12. Some of the vacancy rate decline may have been due to reductions in demand elasticity via their effect on equilibrium vacancies. However, since only the change in such vacancies is likely to be included in the overall rate reported, a decline of the size which was observed (i.e., from approximately 20% to 10%) might be taken as evidence that supply increased relative to demand.

rates—already low in comparison with those for other forms of higher education—will fall.[13]

The only built-in stabilizer—if, in fact, there is one—is the virtual impossibility of pinpointing the loans and scholarships so that they will go to marginal rather than nonmarginal entrants. It is most likely that this aid will not go primarily to marginal entrants, at least until the needs of nonmarginal students have been satisfied. Consequently, very large sums of money may have to be awarded before any appreciable fraction is made available to students who would not otherwise have applied to nursing schools. It is impossible to predict whether Congress will be willing to appropriate sufficient funds to move beyond this threshold level of student support. However, even if Congress is unwilling to appropriate these large sums, it is predictable that the annual increase in graduates will, nonetheless, rise above the present trend. Very few, if any, nonmarginal entrants will be turned away either because financial support could not be secured or because a vacant first-year position was unavailable. Of those who are admitted, practically none will have to drop out owing to financial difficulties; and most schools can be expected to increase their efforts to reduce attrition attributable to other causes as well.

Formulating a comprehensive policy

Clearly, the groundwork has been laid for an increase in the supply of nurses—the effects of which will be with us for many years to come. While there is still time, a major effort should be undertaken to predict the likely consequences of the forces which have been set in motion. Only when this has been done will it be possible to develop a *comprehensive, national policy on nursing*.

Such a policy requires that consideration be given to the demand as well as the supply side of the market. Recent developments point up the importance of making anticipated demand an integral part of the process by which federal priorities for nursing are established. The so-called shortage of nurses has diminished in both economic and needs terms. The observed improvement was brought about not by a large-scale increase in the existing supply of nurses, but, rather, by separately conceived and implemented policies which raised the demand for medical care and, thus, indirectly the *demand* for nurses.

---

13. If this is brought about via better screening of applicants, student counseling, tutorial programs and the like, no adverse effects on quality are likely. However, if standards are lowered in order to graduate all (or nearly all) entrants, this aspect of the legislation could have serious negative implications for quality.

What will happen when these forces interact with the supply increases that the federal nurse training legislation was designed to produce? Although we do not yet know the full answer to this vital question, we do have some preliminary forecasts. Initial simulation experiments performed using the econometric model that I mentioned earlier indicated that an increase in annual nursing school graduations of the magnitude proposed by the SGCGN would have overwhelmed the effects of Medicare-Medicaid on the demand for nurses. Under these conditions, a drastic reduction in the growth rate of nurses' salaries would have occurred. The reduction, in turn, would have lowered the average labor force participation rate, but not sufficiently to prevent the nurse shortage from becoming a surplus (i.e., serious unemployment among nurses would have developed).

While this forecast does not represent the only possible outcome, it does serve to illustrate the basic point that national policy with respect to the supply of nurses should not continue to be developed with little regard for the demand side of the market. The error in seeking to set nurse manpower goals on the basis of needs is that not enough consideration may be given to the problem of converting such needs into effective demand. Continuation of large subsidies for nurse training without adequate consideration for the employment prospects of the resulting graduates will almost certainly worsen, rather than improve, conditions in the market for nurses.

THE ROLE OF ORGANIZED MEDICINE IN DETERMINING OUR HEALTH CARE SYSTEM

REUBEN A. KESSEL

I want to talk about two related topics: first, the role of the American Medical Association (AMA) in determining the rate of output of physicians and, as a consequence, the current supply of physicians, and, second, the role of organized medicine—that is, the AMA—in circumscribing the choice of contractual relationships between physicians and their patients. Because it is my thesis that the famous Flexner report of 1910[1] constituted the key to achieving control over the output of physicians by the AMA, a substantial portion of this lecture is devoted to this report and its implications for understanding of how our society produces physicians.

The Role of the AMA in Determining
the Supply of Physicians

The history of public intervention in the market for medical services can be conveniently divided into two periods. The earlier begins with the publication of the Flexner report and ends with the conclusion of World War II. During this period, public intervention in the market for medical services had its principal effect on the supply of physicians' services. Organized medicine—again, the AMA—using powers delegated by state

NOTE: This lecture was drawn substantially from the author's article, "The A.M.A. and the Supply of Physicians," which was part of a symposium on "Health Care: Part I" and appeared in *Law and Contemporary Problems* 35 (Spring 1970), published by the Duke University School of Law, Durham, North Carolina, copyright 1970, 1971 by Duke University; the lecture is printed here by permission of Duke University.

1. Abraham Flexner, *Medical Education in the United States and Canada,* A Report to the Carnegie Foundation for the Advancement of Teaching (New York: By the Foundation, 1910). Hereinafter cited as the Flexner report.

governments, reduced the output of doctors by making the graduates of some medical schools ineligible to be examined for licensure and by reducing the output of schools that continued to produce eligible graduates. This led to the demise of the schools producing ineligible graduates, since training doctors was the reason for their existence. For the surviving schools, the costs of producing doctors increased enormously.

The later period, which begins with the end of World War II and continues to the present, may be characterized as a period when governmental intervention, through programs such as Kerr-Mills, Medicaid, and Medicare, operated to increase the demand for the services of physicians.

The Flexner report

The Flexner report has been hailed, even by critics of the AMA, as an action by the AMA in the public interest. For example, Dr. John H. Knowles, who was head of perhaps the most prestigious hospital in the United States, Massachusetts General Hospital, has said:

> At the turn of the century, the AMA stood at the forefront of progressive thinking and socially responsible action. Its members had been leaders in forming much-needed public health departments in the States during the last half of the nineteenth century. It formed a Council on Medical Education in 1904 and immediately began an investigation of proprietary medical schools. Because of its success in exposing intolerable conditions in these schools, the Carnegie Foundation, at the AMA's request, commissioned Abraham Flexner to study the national scene. His report in 1910 drove proprietary interests out of medical education, and established it as a full university function with standards for admission, curriculum development, and clinical teaching. Our present system of medical education, essentially unchanged since the Flexner (and AMA) revolution—and acknowledging its current defects—was accomplished through the work of the AMA. Surely this contribution was and is one of its finest in the public interest.[2]

This interpretation of history is going to be challenged. I am going to provide an interpretation which says that the success of the Flexner-AMA revolution accounts for the current scarcity of physicians.

The decline in the number of medical schools and in the output of physicians as a consequence of the Flexner report has been amply documented. Shryock interprets the history of medical education during the period from 1870 to 1910 as a struggle between existing practitioners, represented by the AMA, and medical educators for control over the out-

2. John H. Knowles, M.D., "Where Doctors Fail," *Saturday Review*, 22 Aug. 1970, pp. 21-22.

put of doctors and hence over the medical schools themselves.[3] The victor in this struggle was the AMA, and its most powerful weapon in the battle was the Flexner report on medical schools, which was undertaken and published under the aegis of the prestigious Carnegie Foundation. This report discredited many medical schools and was instrumental in establishing the AMA's wholly owned subdivision, the American Association of Medical Colleges, as the arbiter of which schools could have their graduates sit for state licensure examinations. The first triumph in this campaign was the elimination of the power of medical schools to license their own graduates. The victory was complete when graduation from a Class A medical school, with the ratings determined by this subdivision of the AMA, became a prerequisite for licensure.[4]

It is my thesis that Flexner and the Carnegie Foundation were, to use the language of the Left of the 1930s, "dupes of the interests." In other words, they unwittingly served the highly parochial interests of organized medicine. Flexner's work consisted of a grand inspection tour of the medical schools of the time—some were evaluated in an afternoon—to determine how they produced their output. His model of how doctors should be produced was the medical school of Johns Hopkins University.[5] There was no attempt to evaluate the schools' graduates; there was no investigation of what they could or could not do. Nor was there any discussion of what a graduate of a medical school *should* be able to do, or of the possibility of raising standards of medical education through stiff licensure examinations. The entire burden of improving standards was to be borne by changes in how doctors should be produced—that is, by how students, facilities, and faculty were to be combined to generate physicians. Flexner implicitly ruled out all production functions other than the one he observed at Johns Hopkins.

It is a paradox that a group ostensibly so concerned with doctors' qualifications to practice medicine as the AMA was, failed to be disturbed by Flexner's lack of qualifications for the task he undertook. Flexner was neither a physician nor a scientist, and he had no qualifications as a medical educator. He had an undergraduate degree in arts from Johns Hopkins and had operated a small, private, and apparently profitable preparatory school in Louisville for fifteen years. It is unlikely, if not in-

3. Richard Harrison Shryock, *Medical Licensing in America: 1650-1965* (Baltimore, Md.: Johns Hopkins Press, 1967), pp. 92-93, 108-9, 113.

4. For a description of the AMA's power over medical schools see Harold Margulies and Lucille Block, *Foreign Medical Graduates in the United States* (Cambridge, Mass.: Harvard University Press, 1969), pp. 25-27, 44-45.

5. See Abraham Flexner, *An Autobiography* (New York: Simon and Schuster, 1960), p. 74.

conceivable, that he would have been accepted in a court of law as an expert witness in the field of medical education before he undertook his study.[6]

Moreover, the AMA had essentially completed the Flexner report before Flexner knew about it, for they had inspected medical schools in 1906-7. When Flexner made his tour N.P. Colwell, the secretary of the AMA's Council on Medical Education at the time, accompanied him in some of his inspections and provided him with the results of the AMA's previous labors.[7] Indeed, Flexner spent many hours at the Chicago headquarters of the AMA. It was clearly recognized that Flexner, or more properly the Carnegie Foundation, had an advantage over the AMA in publishing an attack on the medical schools of the time, because the Carnegie Foundation was comparatively invulnerable to a charge of self-interest. "If we could obtain the publication and approval of our work by the Carnegie Foundation for the Advancement of Teaching, it would assist materially in securing the results we were attempting to bring about," to quote an important member of the AMA establishment.[8] So, what you find in Flexner's book is really the work of the AMA which had already been completed, but never published. You can, therefore, raise legitimate questions as to who should be regarded as the author of the Flexner book.

It is a very interesting book, and I strongly recommend that you take a look at it sometime. It is a book that everybody quotes but no one reads, and it deserves to be read. It is really not a book about medicine at all. It is a book about economics, but unfortunately most of the economics is wrong. The book really deals with justifying the restriction on output. It is fascinating reading because Flexner talks about exactly the converse of the situation we have today. He will say, "Now here is this poor, miserable town of 1,500 souls, and they have three doctors. Now how can three doctors make an honest living in this poor, miserable town of 1,500 souls? There isn't enough business for them. One doctor would be plenty for this town." He then invokes Gresham's law by contending that poor doctors are driving good doctors out of business. But he invokes this law incorrectly, because Gresham's law depends on prices being fixed and there is no fixing of prices here.

6. Flexner, *Autobiography*, pp. 78, 79. Significantly, Flexner's brother, who became a very distinguished physician, graduated from a school put out of business.

7. The AMA's Council on Medical Education rated 82 schools Class A in 1906; Flexner rated only 72 schools that high a few years later.

8. Arthur Dean Bevan, "Cooperation in Medical Education and Medical Service," *Journal of the American Medical Association* 90 (1928):1173, 1175.

Consequences of implementing the Flexner report

As a result of the implementation of the Flexner report, medical education became considerably more expensive and exhibited relatively little variation from school to school. The implementation of Flexner's recommendations made medical schools as alike as peas in a pod. In their first year, medical students almost invariably took anatomy, biochemistry, and physiology; in the second, microbiology, pathology, and pharmacology. The next two years consisted of supervised contacts with patients in the major clinical specialties of a teaching hospital. This training pattern was often written into state laws.[9] To this day, there probably is less variation in medical training than in almost any other field.

In addition, experimentation in the training of physicians was sharply reduced until relatively recently. As a result, there was a hiatus of over forty years in the search for better curricula and teaching methods, and in the utilization of the talents of scientists outside medical schools for the training of physicians. It is only in the decade of the 1960s that the fetters imposed by the Flexner report have been loosened. As a consequence, medical education is currently in a state of flux, and the number of electives open to medical students has increased enormously. The economic cost of acquiring the MD degree has started to decrease because medical schools have relaxed their requirement of a bachelor's degree as a condition for admission. Moreover, as a result of student pressure, medical schools have increased their willingness to substitute undergraduate courses for preclinical courses.

A little-recognized consequence of the Flexner report was its effect on the frequency of Negro doctors in the population and on the number of Negro medical schools. Not only were Flexner's views on medical education for Negroes patronizing per se ("A well-taught Negro sanitarian will be immensely useful; an essentially untrained Negro wearing an M.D. degree is dangerous"; "the practice of the Negro doctor will be limited to his own race. . . ."),[10] but as a result of his endeavors and the AMA's the number of medical schools declined from 162 in 1906 to 69 in 1944, with the number of Negro medical schools dropping from 7 to 2, and the number of students admitted to the surviving schools decreased. According to Census figures, the frequency of Negro physicians among all physicians, which had increased sharply between 1900 and 1910 (from 1.3

9. *The Crisis in Medical Services and Medical Education,* Report on an exploratory conference, sponsored by the Commonwealth Fund and the Carnegie Corporation of New York, Fort Lauderdale, Fla., Feb. 1966, p. 7.

10. Flexner report, p. 180.

percent to 2.0 percent), leveled off afterwards. In the absence of Flexner's or more properly the AMA's repression of medical schools, one would have expected the frequency of Negro physicians to rise as the Negro's educational disadvantages were overcome. The Negro's problem of obtaining medical education was intensified by the development of intern and residency programs, because for purely racial reasons many hospitals refused to hire Negroes for their house staffs. The usual argument was that white patients, particularly obstetrical patients, do not wish to be treated by Negro doctors.

Not by chance, 1910 was also a high-water mark for women physicians. Despite the general trend of more women entering the business world, their number in medicine was somewhat smaller (8,810) in 1940 than it had been in 1910.[11]

For those interested in the motive of the AMA in seeking control over medical schools, an unambiguous answer was provided by Bevan, the former head of the AMA's Council on Medical Education:

> In this rapid elevation of the standard of medical education. . .with the reduction of the number of medical schools from 160 to eighty, there occurred a marked reduction in the number of medical students and medical graduates. We had anticipated this and felt that this was a desirable thing. We had. . .a great oversupply of poor mediocre practitioners.[12]

Shryock is a little more circumspect:

> Competing within a free economy they observed that the scientific motive for educational reform coincided with their own professional ambitions. They became increasingly aware that too many schools were turning out too many graduates to make practice profitable.[13]

The advent of licensure and the closing of those medical schools that failed to meet AMA standards were of course justified as a measure to protect the public from the ministrations of unqualified or incompetent physicians. But when higher standards were imposed, there was no immediate improvement in quality of practice, since the graduates of those medical schools which were put out of business continue to practice. As is commonplace whenever licensure is imposed upon a previously unlicensed activity or new standards are imposed, grandfather clauses protected the rights of existing physicians to continue to practice medicine regardless of the adequacy of their training. Indeed, as late as 1942 or 1943 there was a medical school put out of business—Middlesex College. Yet, I imagine,

11. Richard Harrison Shryock, "Women in American Medicine," *Journal of the American Medical Women's Association* 5 (1950):371, 377.

12. Bevan, *Journal of the American Medical Association* 90 (1928):1176.

13. Shyrock, *Medical Licensing in America,* p. 57.

there are probably some graduates of Middlesex Medical College practicing in western Massachusetts to this day, and it was very heavily represented among practitioners in western Massachusetts for quite some time. Hence, the effects of the change in training standards for physicians could not have been realized until many years after Flexner's work.

The effects of the restriction on opportunities to study medicine in this country were particularly oppressive to Jews and Negroes.[14] The AMA had conducted another survey of medical schools, the Weiskotten survey, following the decrease in demand for medical services caused by the Great Depression of the 1930s. This resulted in a cutback in admissions to medical schools. I have some figures on that which show that Negroes and Jews were cut back about 30 percent, while the overall reduction was about 17 percent.[15] And circumstantial evidence indicates that females also bore a disproportionate share of the reduction in admissions.

As a result of the Flexner report and the restriction of opportunities for medical education in this country, foreign medical schools, particularly in the late 1930s, were deluged by American applicants. If one divides graduate training in U.S. institutions into the categories of business administration, agriculture, education, engineering, physical and natural sciences, economics, and medicine, then foreign enrollments in U.S. institutions exceed U.S. enrollments in foreign institutions by a wide margin for all fields but one—medicine. Americans studying abroad range from one-fourth to one-thirtieth of foreigners studying in the United States for six of the seven categories. But the ratio of Americans studying medicine abroad to foreigners studying medicine in the United States exceeded three-to-one for the year 1966.[16] Apparently the restriction of opportunities in this country continues to affect the number of Americans studying medicine abroad.

And the last time I checked into it, something like 10 percent of all Americans studying medicine are going to foreign medical schools. It is a paradox that we provide all these opportunities for people if they want to study to become insurance agents, real estate salesmen, etc. In most cases the state is ready to pour money into training people for many different kinds of occupations. Yet for medicine there do not seem to be enough opportunities for Americans to study medicine in this country.

14. See A. Alchian and R. Kessel, "Competition, Monopoly, and the Pursuit of Money," in National Bureau of Economic Research, *Aspects of Labor Economics* (Princeton, N.J.: Princeton University Press, 1962), p. 157.

15. See Jacob A. Goldberg, "Jews in the Medical Profession—A National Survey," *Jewish Social Studies* 1 (1939):332.

16. See Institute on International Education, *Open Doors* (New York: By the Institute, 1967); American Council on Higher Education, *A Fact Book on Higher Education* (Washington, D.C.: By the Council, 1967), looseleaf.

Educational cost and physicians' fees

I want to turn to the question of educational cost and physician fees. It is, of course, a well-known axiom that a rise in quality requires an increase in price. And an increase in price implies an increase in efforts to economize on a resource that has become more scarce. Hence, improved quality implies a greater effort to economize on physicians' services. What this means specifically is that people tend to substitute self-diagnosis and self-treatment for the services of a physician. This tendency manifests itself at the onset of an illness or suspected illness, when going to a physician possibly is deferred until the symptoms become alarming. Consequently, increasing the quality of physicians' skill does not necessarily imply that the quality of medical care that the public receives as a whole also improves, since the public receives a mixture of professional attention and self-treatment.

The foregoing argument about the effect improvement in quality has on price has been countered with the argument that higher standards protect all of the public. Those too poor "to afford" good medical care, so the argument runs, would and do receive it free. Money is not a barrier to receiving medical services. Since these views have received wide acceptance by both the public and economists, they deserve attention.

Economists as well as other observers have inferred, incorrectly, that if care is provided by physicians at no out-of-pocket or pecuniary cost to the patient, an act of charity has occurred. They have forgotten that transactions at a zero price can be economically profitable for everyone involved. Most of the so-called free care that was traditionally provided by the medical profession fell into three categories: (1) work done by neophytes or beginners, particularly in the surgical specialties, who wanted to develop their skills and who require practice; (2) services of experienced physicians in free clinics who wished to develop new skills or maintain existing skills so they could better serve their private, paying patients; and (3) services to maintain staff and medical appointments, which are of great value financially. The advent of Medicare and Medicaid has reduced the availability of "charity" patients, who, to employ the language of the medical profession, were used as "teaching material," and has led to readjustments in training procedures, particularly for residents.[17]

To see that the free care argument can not be taken seriously, all one need do is examine the relationship of infant mortality to income. The infant mortality rate is highly sensitive to the absence or presence of medical

17. Citizens' Commission on Graduate Medical Education, *The Graduate Education of Physicians* (Chicago: American Medical Association, 1966), pp. 75, 77. (The Millis Report.)

care, particularly prenatal care. Clearly Negroes have lower incomes and higher infant mortality rates than whites; they have not been provided with enough free care to offset the effects of income differences. Moreover, infant mortality rates in the United States do not compare favorably with a number of European countries, including some that extensively use midwives. Charity, with or without quotation marks, can not be regarded as an important means for offsetting the effects of restriction on entry into the practice of medicine.

The argument that restrictions on entry and licensure has raised standards of medical practice has great appeal and acceptance. Unfortunately, there does not appear to be any empirical study available to support this view, and it is striking that organized medicine has not investigated the effects of licensure on the quality of care in the community. The usual statement one hears is that Americans have the best medical care in the world. In my view if the contention were "the most expensive," it would probably be easier to buttress.

Licensure as a barrier to entry

Many distinguished writers, some in the field of political economy, have argued for free entry into the practice of medicine—for giving the public freedom to choose anyone as a physician without constraint by the state. This view is evident in the famous letter of Adam Smith to Cullen[18] and in a letter of William James to his fellow physicians in Boston.[19] It is also the position of my colleague, Professor Milton Friedman.[20] This view was expressed as well by Samuel Clemens as by anyone. When he found out that MDs were trying to put osteopaths out of business in his state, he said,

> I don't know that I cared much about these osteopaths until I heard you were going to drive them out of the State; but since I heard that I haven't been able to sleep.
> Now, what I contend is that my body is my own, at least I have always so regarded it. If I do harm through my experimenting with it, it is I who suffer, not the State.[21]

18. Manfred S. Guttmacher, "The Views of Adam Smith on Medical Education," *Bulletin of Johns Hopkins Hospital* 47 (1930):164, 171.

19. Henry James, ed., *The Letters of William James* 2 (Boston: Atalantic Monthly Press, 1920), pp. 66 ff.

20. See Milton Friedman, *Capitalism and Freedom* (Chicago: University of Chicago Press, 1962), p. 149.

21. See Andrews, "Medical Practice and the Law," *Forum* 31(1901): 542, 547.

By using licensure as a barrier to entry, our society has, to a large extent, abandoned freedom of choice of physicians. It is pertinent to turn to an examination of this professed policy of protecting the public from making a poor choice of physicians. How consistent has organized medicine been in adhering to the implications of its argument about protecting the public from incompetent doctors?

1. There is a substantial body of evidence that there has been discrimination in terms of race, creed, and color in admission to medical schools. This discrimination became especially severe when there was a cutback in the production of doctors in the mid-1930s as a result of the onset of the Great Depression, and Negroes and Jews (and possibly women) seem to have borne a disproportionate share of the reduction in admissions to medical schools. Clearly, the cutback in output can not be justified as an effort to maintain quality of medical care, since discrimination in terms of race, creed, and color reduces the quality of the student population in medical schools.

2. When higher standards were instituted, they were not made applicable to existing practitioners. Hence, it was future and not current generations that would benefit from any improvement of standards. Yet, so far as the public is concerned, there are no grounds for distinguishing between mistreatment by recent, as distinguished from less recent, graduates of medical schools.

3. There is no reexamination procedure for doctors. Once a doctor wins a license to practice, it is almost never revoked unless he is convicted of law-breaking. It is pertinent to ask why holders of automobile drivers' licenses are subject to reexamination and holders of licenses to practice medicine are not. Is medicine less important? Why are commercial airline pilots subject to reexamination, but physicians are not? Clearly, to be consistent in one's concern about maintaining high quality, there should be a periodic reexamination of physicians with recertification to insure that physicians keep current on what constitutes good practice.

4. Politics has been intertwined with decisions that should be based on quality considerations alone. An important instance has been the requirement that a doctor be a member of his county medical society in order to qualify for membership in a specialty board. Obviously, membership in the AMA has nothing to do with a doctor's qualifications for membership on a specialty board.

5. Doctors run most hospitals in the sense that they have de facto control over staff appointments. For most medical specialists, being on the staff of a hospital is imperative for successful practice. Yet appointment decisions are not based solely on considerations of skill and talent, but are similar to admissions procedures to a country club—race, religion, family, type of practice, and so forth are often important.

6. Within the medical profession there exists great internal solidarity and cohesion. This is much stronger in medicine than in a field characterized by free entry, such as the profession of economics. As a consequence, there tends to be a closed loop of referrals of patients from one doctor to another, and patients are unable to form effective coalitions with doctors in buying the services of other doctors. It is very difficult to obtain the judgment of the profession about comparative rankings of doctors in particular fields and parts of the country. The difficulty of obtaining doctors to testify as expert witnesses for plaintiffs in malpractice suits is so widespread that lawyers used to assert that a "conspiracy of silence" existed. For these reasons, the incentive to produce quality work and to develop an outstanding reputation is not so strong as it would be in a field in which such information could be more easily obtained.

For all these reasons, it is difficult to credit seriously the protestations of the medical profession that its concern in establishing control over medical schools was quality. Improvements in the quality of the graduates of medical schools probably did occur. Yet, if the experience of law schools is relevant, improvements undoubtedly would have occurred without the efforts of the organized profession. It was this promised improvement in the quality of graduates that sold the public and legislators on giving regulatory powers to organized medicine. Economic gains to the medical profession resulting from restriction on output constitutes a better explanation of the shutting down of medical schools than does the desire to raise standards.

Even if one prefers to accept the view that those responsible for restricting the output of physicians were not economically motivated, however, one can hardly deny that the output of doctors has in fact been unresponsive to market forces. The increases in demand for medical services, particularly those brought about by Medicare and Medicaid, have had relatively little impact on the number of doctors graduated by American medical schools. As a consequence, the prices of physicians' services have risen dramatically, and there has been a shift of medical resources away from the population at large and toward the beneficiaries of Medicare and Medicaid. This analysis suggests that the proposed measures to increase the demand for medical care, such as the extension of Medicare to segments of the population under age sixty-five, would not increase the availability of physicians to the population in general and, if anything, would be more likely to reduce their availability. That is, if you feel there might be a backward-bending supply curve for physicians, it could be argued that the rise in price would decrease the availability of medical care in the population.

Innovation in medical education

Now I would like to turn to the question of innovation in medical education. The current problem of the relative scarcity of physicians had its origin in the victory of organized medicine over educators in their battle for control of medical education. Educators have a much stronger interest in producing doctors than has organized medicine, and if given the opportunity educators would act to make the supply of physicians responsive to consumer desires. Unfortunately, the options open to medical educators have been narrower than is true in most academic disciplines.

To see what can be done to increase output, it is useful to contrast post- with pre-MD training. There seems to be an abundance of facilities in the United States for post-MD training. Approved spaces in hospitals for post-MD training—that is, training more advanced than medical school training—exceed the annual output of American medical schools by quite a wide margin. As a result, one finds large numbers of non-American graduates of foreign medical schools taking intern and residency training in this country. Despite these imports, many unfilled vacancies exist. Intern and residency programs have never been regarded as difficult to expand. Approved residencies in hospitals increased 600 percent between 1940 and 1960, while the output of medical graduates rose only 35 percent. These advanced programs are under the aegis of hospitals rather than medical schools, although university-affiliated hospitals are overrepresented in most post-MD training. It is an educational anomaly that the more advanced the training, the greater the availability of facilities, and that the more specialized and advanced training often takes place outside medical schools.

Why should the facilities for post-MD training be disproportionately large relative to pre-MD training? An explanation of this phenomenon rests on the hypothesis that there exist economic benefits to the medical profession from post-MD training that are virtually nonexistent from pre-

MD training. The interns and residents of a hospital, the so-called house staff, are hospital employees and a large part of their duties consists of aiding the attending staff in the care of their patients. Despite the time costs involved in instruction, the attending staff can gain time in the long run by delegating duties to the house staff that they would otherwise have to perform for themselves. Hence, doctors that are members of the attending staff of a hospital with a large intern and residency training program have an important competitive advantage stemming from their lower costs of producing patient care. Needless to say, the prized positions for attending staffs are in hospitals with extensive intern and residency training programs. Consequently, the staffs of hospitals without educational programs push hard to obtain such programs. No economic benefit of a comparable magnitude exists in the case of pre-MD programs. It is true that third- and fourth-year medical students have some value around a hospital, but they are not worth as much as post-MD students. First- and second-year medical students are a dead weight with respect to instructional costs and, in the past, have provided no useful output in a hospital. Indeed, because of small classes and expensive facilities, costs of instruction for the first two years of medical school are relatively high.

The foregoing suggests that the bottleneck in medical education is the first two years of medical school when, under the Flexner curricula, medical students take their so-called basic science courses. Serious questions can be raised as to whether or not these courses ought to be taught in a medical school at all. They are relatively elementary and are often taught by faculties that are undistinguished when compared with the biological and physical science faculties in many universities. Let us take a couple of specific examples. I doubt that the people teaching basic science at most medical schools within the United States are on par with the people teaching the same courses, say, at Cal Tech or MIT, institutions that have very distinguished faculties but no medical schools. Moreover, many medical students have already completed some of these courses in their premedical studies and find ordinary medical school teaching duplicative as well as inferior and, hence, a waste of time. It is difficult to understand why medical schools could not divest themselves of this elementary instruction and concentrate on their field of comparative advantage—clinical teaching, both pre- and post-MD.

If medical schools were to divest themselves of responsibility for preclinical teaching of basic sciences, then a number of interesting developments would follow: the resources of institutions which do not have medical schools but do have outstanding science departments could play a role in training physicians, and the role of the science departments in schools with medical schools could be more active; the preclinical years of medical training could become part of undergraduate study, thereby shortening the period of production of doctors by two years and effecting an enormous reduction in the costs of producing MDs; and finally, the resources liberated from training in basic sciences could be employed to expand the number trained by medical schools and to increase the quality of post-MD training, which is now largely outside the province of existing medical schools and almost wholly didactic.

The currently important social problem is how to make medical schools responsive to the demands of the market for physicians. One solution is to enlist the aid of the nonmedical sector of the educational establishment in providing basic science training and to utilize the resources liberated in medical schools for expansion of enrollments of third- and fourth-year medical students. However, this is but one suggestion in a field of education that has been relatively stagnant for many years.

An unfortunate heritage of Flexner's work is the overspecification of how doctors are to be produced. Consequently, we have not had the natural experimentation in educational techniques that otherwise would have been available. If Flexner had specified what knowledge and capabilities a physician should have and had given medical educators the freedom to search for efficient techniques for producing the desired results, we would currently know a great deal more about how to produce physicians efficiently. Undoubtedly we also would have many more physicians, because the costs of their production would have been considerably lower and because production would not have been cut back in the 1930s. Medical education has been made artificially expensive because of the overspecification of how it was to be produced, particularly (but not exclusively) during the first two years of medical school. As a result, many writers on the subject explicitly or implicitly accept the view that medical education is extremely costly, just as if this were a natural constant like the speed of light.

The search for efficiency in medical education could be stimulated by opening state licensure examinations and/or national boards to all applicants without concern over how they received their medical education or the rating, if any, of the schools they attended. To insure that this examination is not used by the medical profession as a barrier to entry, it should bear a reasonable resemblance to the examination that existing practitioners would be asked, from time to time, to pass. Such a move could increase both the output of physicians and their quality. It could enable the community to move closer to economic efficiency in the production of physicians, since both quality and quantity could be increased without any change in aggregate expenditures.

The Effect of the AMA on the
Marketing of Medical Services

My final point concerns the role that the AMA has played in health care delivery. I contend that rigidity in medical education has been matched, if not surpassed, by rigidity in the marketing of medical services. The AMA long ago discovered that fee-for-service is the ideal way of marketing medical care. Moreover, so great was its confidence in the correctness of this view that the Association opposed any other method of marketing medical care in order to prevent less intelligent brethren from falling into error. This opposition took two forms: working for legislation to prohibit alternative methods of marketing medical care, and refusing hospital staff appointments to physicians associated with such unapproved methods.

More specifically, the AMA, or organized medicine, bitterly opposed comprehensive prepaid group medical plans, or HMOs as they came to be known, such as Kaiser, Ross-Loos, Group Health, and HIP. Plans of this type are illegal in seventeen, or about one-third, of the states in the United States. Where they are legal, nevertheless they are opposed, and the chief weapon used to fight these plans was to deny access to hospitals for patients of physicians in such plans. As a consequence, the AMA was prosecuted under the Sherman Act in Washington, D.C., and under state antitrust laws elsewhere. Physicians without a taste for martyrdom were deterred from joining such programs, and there is little doubt that the commitment of organized medicine to fee-for-service has inhibited the search for and experimentation with alternatives to this method of marketing medical care. Hence, as with medical education, there is less experimental knowledge about the marketing of medical services than would have been available if organized medicine were less powerful and there were more freedom to innovate.

Nevertheless, not all prepaid group plans have been aborted, and much can be learned from those that have been born, and especially from the ones that have survived to maturity. One of the most interesting aspects of these plans is that under them surgeons are less numerous and surgery less frequent than in the usual fee-for-service practice.

The lower frequency of surgery for prepaid group plan members has been explained as a consequence of differences in economic incentives. In comprehensive prepaid plans, the costs of a marginal unit of surgery (hospitalization and surgical service) are borne by the plan, with the marginal revenue from this surgery being zero. By contrast, under fee-for-service the marginal revenue of an additional unit of surgery is positive to the surgeon, since he receives a surgical fee; hospital costs are borne by the patient or his insurer. Consequently, it has been argued that some surgery is performed under fee-for-service that would not have been performed under prepaid medical care. An alternative interpretation of these same findings is that members of prepaid plans go outside their plans to buy surgery, forgoing rights to surgery at zero marginal costs in order to shop at positive marginal costs in the fee-for-service medical market. While I think that this might happen in some cases, I really find it hard to believe that that is the case generally. If patients are going to do that, why should they go on the plan in the first place?

Another aspect of this problem, which has not been explored in the literature, is that the individual surgeon in comprehensive prepaid plans apparently undertakes more surgery per month or per year than the surgeon in fee-for-service arrangements. When the number of surgical procedures per surgeon is aggregated by using Blue Cross or Medicare fee schedules as index numbers, one finds that this total measure is greater for the prepaid plan surgeons than for the fee-for-service surgeons. To understand why this should be the case, it is helpful to examine the anomalous characteristics of the surgical market.

The consumer enters into virtually no other contracts involving expenditures as large as those involved in surgical fees without knowing the specific price before his purchase. Yet patients almost never discuss fees with their surgeons before operations; one in twenty would probably be a high estimate of the portion of patients who know their surgeon's fee before they commit themselves to surgery. This alone suggests that surgery is not characterized by a high degree of price competition; price wars are undoubtedly more common in other fields.

Systematic price discrimination in the provision of surgical services is further evidence of the absence of price competition, and it is made possible by organized medicine's control over access to hospital beds. There is no comparable control over fees for office visits, and consumer knowledge of the prices for office visits is considerably greater.

A consequence of the absence of price competition is that the rate of exchange of surgical for nonsurgical services in the market fails to reflect the rate of exchange in production. Therefore, too many physicians are attracted into surgery, and they are apt to be underemployed compared to physicians in the nonsurgical specialties. This misallocation has been aggravated by the onset of Medicare and Medicaid, which in general have more generous surgical fee schedules than Blue Cross, and it is not unknown for patients to be charged surgical fees as much as 50 percent greater than the Medicare rate, which is supposed to reflect the prevailing rate in the community. Medicare, which has increased the ability of some members of the community to pay for surgery, has consequently increased the price of surgery.

A great virtue of prepaid group medical plans is that the marginal cost of the time of surgeons is lower to such plans than it is to the public. The price per surgical procedure under fee-for-service is regulated; the price of a surgeon's time to a plan that will convert this time into surgical procedures is not. Hence, prepaid plans represent a means of cutting prices for surgical services. Alternatively, prepaid plans constitute means for buying surgical and nonsurgical services at prices that reflect their relative costs of production.

Many writers have found fault with our medical care delivery system on the grounds that it is a "cottage industry," characterized by a large number of small firms which, in their judgment, are operating at less than optimal size. One of the striking pieces of evidence obtained from our experience with comprehensive prepaid group medical plans, which are relatively large-scale enterprises, is that advertising is crucial to getting started and to generating sufficient volume to justify attempts to achieve scale economies. Many of the successful and unsuccessful prepaid plans ran into trouble with organized medicine because they advertised. The AMA usually roundly condemns advertising as being unethical, although it has never made clear why advertising should not be permitted. It appears that freedom to advertise is important if we want to encourage innovation in the marketing of medical care.

Conclusion

In summary, the production (education) of physicians and the delivery of health care have both suffered from the inability of institutions and individuals to innovate because of the restraints imposed by organized medicine. In the education of physicians, it was a mistake to specify how physicians were to be produced instead of specifying what the product should be and allowing schools to compete in efficiently producing that product. State licensure examinations or the national board examinations constitute an appropriate vehicle for specifying what physicians can be expected to do. Medical schools should be free to decide how to produce whatever it is that constitutes a physician without intervention by the state or the AMA.

Similarly, in the case of medical care delivery, individuals and groups should be free to innovate alternative delivery systems. There is no case for sanctifying fee-for-service and making prepaid plans illegal. Nor is there any good reason for prohibiting advertising by physicians.

In the decade of the 1960's, and particularly in the last five years, the AMA began openly to admit that a shortage of doctors exists. Many new medical schools have been started, restrictions on the use of paramedical personnel have been relaxed, and some innovations in the medical curricula have reduced the time it takes to produce an MD. This behavior is subject to two interpretations—either (1) the AMA has changed its spots or (2) the times are embarrassingly good financially for the medical profession and, hence, a more relaxed attitude is appropriate. The history of the AMA suggests that the latter interpretation is the more correct. During the prosperity of the late 1920s, the AMA was less restrictive than it was during the Great Depression.

It is important to remember that, whatever the times, the AMA has an inevitable conflict of interests. It has presumed to represent simultaneously both the public—in maintaining standards for the production of physicians and in determining the quantity to be produced—and the medical profession, the purveyors of medical services. In other words, the AMA represents both the buyers and the sellers of physician services. Given this anomalous position, it is difficult to believe that the AMA will ever permit the production of physicians in the numbers that the public is willing to support with its patronage. Consequently, the AMA's power to determine output via the rating of medical schools should be withdrawn, and graduation from an AMA-approved medical school should not be a condition for admission to licensure examinations.

It is important to remember that physicians, not Congressmen, produce medical care. To extend Medicare to include everyone, as some of the National Health Insurance proposals have suggested, would increase the demand for medical care and probably reduce the availability of physicians. The problem of supply that exists in medicine is largely a consequence of the severe restriction in the output of physicians that was caused by the AMA and abetted, probably unwittingly, by Flexner and the Carnegie Foundation. Hence, the solution to our problems regarding the supply of physicians lies in increasing the output and in making the number of physicians in the community responsive to the desires of the community. To accomplish this goal, the AMA should be stripped of its power to control the education of physicians.

WHAT KIND OF HEALTH INSURANCE
SHOULD THE UNITED STATES CHOOSE?

HERBERT E. KLARMAN

The question posed, "What kind of health insurance should the United States choose?" is not altogether new in this country. It was widely discussed around 1915, in the 1930s, and most recently in the late 1940s. It is being asked again in 1974, after 45 years of experience with voluntary health insurance and almost ten years of experience with Medicare for people aged 65 and over.

We know more about health insurance today than we knew in 1948, the last time national health insurance was a serious issue in this country. We know more about what it is likely to accomplish, because some of these effects—good, bad, or neutral—have already occurred. We also know more about what health insurance is not likely to bring about, because some problems in the health field appear to be rather impervious to financial incentives, at least in the doses which we are accustomed to administering.

Experience to date

The recent return of national health insurance to our active political agenda is perhaps as much attributable to the past successes of voluntary health insurance and of Medicare as it is to their failures and the failings of a major companion public program for the poor, Medicaid. To date the several programs jointly have demonstrated the practicability for this country of large-scale purchase of health services by so-called third parties. Thus, when government becomes a major source of financial support, it is no longer deemed necessary, as it was in England after World War II, to nationalize the hospitals and put their medical specialists on salary. As intended under health insurance, the burden of major illness has been mitigated for many, while there has been an increase in the use of services by the poor and the near poor, relative to use by the rest of the population. Most providers of service have prospered financially, even as they have been left undisturbed professionally and organizationally. Either some of the fears concerning governmental interference in the practice of medicine that were voiced by opponents of health insurance were groundless, or the very expression of these fears and the reassurances elicited in response combined to deflect what would have been a different course of events.

On the other side of the ledger are some unintended, certainly unexpected, side effects of health insurance, mostly adverse. Hospital use has steadily increased in step with bed supply. After World War II, hospital costs rose year by year, as wages were periodically allowed to catch up with those in other industries, as labor productivity gains continued to lag behind those in the rest of the economy, and as scientific progress served to create more complex care. After 1965, when Medicare for the elderly and Medicaid for the poor and the near poor were enacted simultaneously, the rate of increase in patient-day cost doubled from 6.5 percent to 13 percent a year. The annual rate of increase in physicians' fees rose to 6 percent after 1965, compared with 3 percent in the preceding five-year period. Fractionation of fees, not reflected in the official Consumer Price Index, served to increase physicians' incomes even more, while physicians sometimes reduced the volume of services rendered. As a result, total expenditures for health services in the United States continued to rise at 10 percent or more a year. This has been true even under Phase IV of the federal Economic Stabilization Program, which has singled out the health services industry for special control measures.[1]

Health services expenditures first rose above 4 percent of the GNP a generation ago. Yet, 4 percent used to be regarded as a universal ceiling above which expenditures for health services would not, and could not, go. The ratio of health services expenditures to the GNP was 5.2 percent in 1960, almost 6 percent in 1965, and 7.7 percent in fiscal year 1973.

An even more striking change in the past decade has been the rise in the proportion of total expenditures paid from public funds. For 15 years the proportion of public to total funds was a stable fraction of one-fourth, but after 1965 the fraction rose abruptly, and today it falls just short of two-fifths. The proportion has been kept down slightly by successive legislative and administrative actions that serve to curtail expenditures under the government programs, especially Medicaid.

In contrast to these substantial changes in total expenditures by type of service (hospital, doctor, and so forth) and in sources of funds, certain

1. Again, the reader will note this paper was given before the May 1974 discontinuation of wage and price controls.—Ed.

organizational and behavioral features and tendencies of the health services system in this country remain unchanged. The 50-year-old trend from general practice to specialty practice in medicine has continued unabated. The workload of hospital emergency departments steadily increases. Geographic maldistribution of health care resources abounds. Long-term care has remained outside the mainstream of medicine, generally rejected by the nonprofit sector.

For many of us, these developments are not attuned to our preferences. Had our preferences prevailed, these long-term tendencies would have been reversed or at least attenuated some time ago. It would take one very far afield to begin to account for their persistence and why they have been able to withstand widespread deploring and constant attack. It is fair to say that none appears to be strongly responsive to financial incentives within the known range of such incentives. Other, nonpecuniary, factors seem to be more important in career choice and location, especially when the level of professional income attained in the health field is high enough.

It seems plausible, then, to posit that a general mechanism for financing services, such as national health insurance, cannot play a substantial part in an effective effort to influence the direction or scope of these behavioral and organizational features of the health services system. Other approaches, such as finely tuned new arrangements for hospital staff appointments for physicians, perhaps changing the geographic origins of some medical students, possibly promoting the growth of the comprehensive health maintenance organizations popularly known as the HMOs, have been suggested as promising devices for alleviating these problems. However, there is no basis in experience in this country or elsewhere for predicting success even if carefully designed schemes were adopted.

Even more insensitive to the type of incentives that national health insurance is likely to embody than are these features of the present health services system (the unabated trend toward specialization, the reliance on emergency care, the geographic maldistribution, and medicine's general neglect of long-term care) are those factors in the environment and individual life style which, under many circumstances, are more important determinants of health status than is medical care. It is necessary to acknowledge the limited nature of a mechanism aimed essentially at financing personal health services.

Despite the intractability of certain problems and their lack of susceptibility to financial incentives, it *is* progress, I believe, to recognize that this country is not at present in the midst of a health crisis. True, the steps that are recommended to deal with a so-called health crisis often seem irrelevant to its manifestations. Nevertheless, it is salubrious to realize that we have sufficient time available to us to review policies and to act on that realization. Today it cannot be said that pressure exists for urgent action on national health insurance because a health crisis requires it. Indeed, it is reassuring to learn that the infant mortality rate in this country has been dropping, that adult heart disease mortality has been declining, and that adult life expectancy has improved appreciably in the past 40-50 years for whites and blacks, males and females. Accordingly, there is time to think about our health services problems and how we might go about alleviating or solving them. There is surely time to appraise the available evidence—whether it derives from experience or from analytical study—and to analyze and weigh alternatives. Where firm evidence is lacking, there is time to take care to design policies that are reversible, if they prove to be in error. There is even time to conduct some modest research studies. Certainly there is time to list and elaborate on a set of criteria for assessing a desirable program of national health insurance and to appraise various proposals in terms of their agreement with such criteria. This last task I take to be the heart of my present assignment.

Criteria for Assessing a National Health Insurance Plan

Against this historical background, and with due recognition of the limitations inherent in a financing mechanism like national health insurance, we turn to the original question, "What kind of health insurance should the United States choose?" My answers to the question will be stated in terms of general principle, but hopefully not in generalities. I intend to be as concrete as possible through elaboration of the argument and by drawing on suitable examples. Although I shall not offer an analysis of individual bills before Congress, the influence of the 1974 Nixon proposal, the Comprehensive Health Insurance Plan, on the issues that I have selected to discuss are undeniable.

I propose, then, to formulate my answers to the question in the form of a set of criteria for assessing whatever national health insurance plan comes before us. Excluded from such an appraisal of national health insurance, it will be understood, are those aspects of the environment and individual life style that exert a highly important effect on health status and those aspects of the health services system which seem rather unresponsive to financial incentives.

I believe that the argument concerning the limited nature of national health insurance as a policy instrument extends to some phenomena which are otherwise closely related to health insurance or prepayment. For example, the close association that has been observed between short-term hospital use and bed supply and summarized under the heading of Roemer's Law, though largely based on the growth of prepayment, may not be reversible through financial actions of a magnitude that are also practicable. For the demand by the patient for hospital care is rather unresponsive to price variation. This is true not only because health insurance has resulted in a low out-of-pocket price, but also because under our system of organization the patient chooses the doctor, who chooses the hospital for him. Moreover, a hospital's financial stability is no longer threatened when high use of its beds is assured. It follows that the only effective remedy for a high level of hospital use is to curtail the supply of beds. A direct order by a duly constituted authority not to add beds, or not to replace existing beds, or even to eliminate certain beds seems necessary. Alternatively, we might conceive of the imposition of drastic financial sanctions far beyond the application of the ordinary financial incentives of a system of prices. However, with these measures we are invoking the instrumentalities of health planning and regulation, not of financing.

In order to ascertain what national health insurance is likely to be capable of accomplishing, it is helpful to return to the first principles of health insurance. The major objective has always been to mitigate the burden of the unexpected and uneven costs of illness on a population by equalizing the burden among its members. This objective is predicated on the assumption that people are risk averters, not gamblers; that they are adverse to large income losses and do not mind small losses at reasonably fair odds. On this basis health insurance constitutes a worthwhile service apart from any other benefits that it may yield, such as facilitating going to the doctor and thus perhaps permitting the early detection of illness or the timely arresting of illness before exacerbation. Nor is it socially disadvantageous if health insurance yields a measure of financial stability to the providers of health services.

Some effects that health insurance produced, such as an increase in health care expenditures, were perhaps not expected. In retrospect, however, it is evident that transferring the financial burden from the ill to the well by charging everybody small sums periodically is bound to raise the total amount devoted to spending on health services. The subsidy granted to employer contributions to health insurance premiums under the individual income tax and the social security tax likewise increases the money pool. The very existence of health insurance apparently yields a measure of assurance to consumers that might lead them to spend more on all health services, insured or otherwise. An increase in the amount of income devoted to a particular service is tantamount to an increase in demand. At a given price, more units are taken or a given volume of services commands a higher price. Whether and when such changes in price or quantity may be deemed excessive is a separate question, one that does not yield unambiguous, meaningful answers.

Importance of universal enrollment

To equalize the financial burden of illness among a population while allowing ready access to care, enrollment must be universal. Medicare comes close to 100 percent enrollment for the aged—persons 65 and over. Voluntary health insurance, though achieving volumes of enrollment beyond all forecasts made by friends and foes alike in the 1930s and 1940s, does not. For the population under age 65 the health insurance enrollment figures are not precisely known. Official estimates from the Social Security Administration vary between 80 and 91 percent for hospital care, which has the largest enrollment among the several objects of health expenditure. Enrollment for physician's services in the hospital is reported to range between 77 and 84 percent of the population under 65. For physician's services outside the hospital, out-of-hospital prescribed drugs, private-duty nursing, and visiting nurse service, the proportion of the population enrolled ranges between 50 and 60 percent, mostly under major medical insurance. It is noteworthy that for in-hospital services the percentage of the population enrolled has been virtually at a plateau since 1967.

It is not evident how much of a deviation from 100 percent enrollment is acceptable in the real world. Certainly, voluntary health insurance is unlikely to reach 100 percent enrollment, even if only because some people are gamblers, willing to take a chance that serious illness will not strike them, while others brought up in the Western tradition count on getting a free ride in case of a medical emergency. But—if it was not clear in the 1940s and 1950s as a matter of logic, it is clear now with our experience under Medicaid—medically indigent persons, once they are ill, are not insurable. And persons who are not yet ill and are not covered by insurance are liable to lose their eligibility for free care when government budgets for health programs are cut back. In places like New York City with a long-time liberal tradition of free care, some persons were worse off after Medicaid was instituted than before. Their condition was further aggravated by the higher prices they were now supposed to pay out-of-pocket.

In sum, it turns out, that under voluntary health insurance the deviation from 100 percent enrollment is appreciable. Thirty or forty years ago, the gap was masked sometimes by the cushioning effect of free or partly free care provided in government hospitals, usually local or federal; in voluntary, nonprofit hospitals subsidized by philanthropic funds; and in private physicians' offices, where a sliding scale of fees applied. In the course of time, the sliding scale has become eroded, owing to its essential incompatability with health insurance (which serves to enhance the patient's ability to pay) and the fact that the philanthropic dollar buys less than formerly.

Local public hospitals, sponsored and operated by municipalities, have become dependent on federal and state funds and are compelled to reduce service when outside funds are cut back. Only the Veterans Administration system, owned and operated by the federal government, has remained intact in size, if not unchanged in program composition. It follows that a given deviation from enrollment of 100 percent of the population in a health insurance plan is a more serious concern today than it would have been a generation ago.

Unless the voluntary nature of health insurance enrollment possesses intrinsic merits that are not discernible to this observer, there are no reasons for departing from the principle of universal enrollment. There may be administrative difficulties that would have to be attended to during the period of transition in implementing such a goal. But the target must not be allowed to recede. Too many workers change jobs, too many people work part time to make health insurance enrollment dependent on permanent, full-time attachment to the labor force. Enrollment, not merely the opportunity to enroll, must be extended to all. Universality of enrollment, then, is the first of the proposed criteria for assessing the merits of a national health insurance plan.

Benefits package

Next to consider is the benefits package. In this country, health insurance benefits have developed unevenly. Coverage of hospital care has always led coverage for other, related services. In consequence, some distortion in use has followed, with the insured service, even when more costly, sometimes substituted for cheaper, uninsured services. It is widely agreed now that a broad package of benefits for related health services is superior to a narrow package.

The exclusion of a nonrelated service, such as long-term care, is less harmful in the context of the benefits package and may be dealt with as a separate issue. Nevertheless the financing of long-term care on a systematic basis has been neglected too long. Usually required as a result of deterioration in health status, long-term care is a service properly encompassed within the health services industry. It may, however, be subject to different conditions of purchase, because it does not fall within the usual orbit of the physician-hospital relationship. Moreover, the components of long-term care are more susceptible to evaluation by the patient and his family than are those of acute medical and hospital care.

In retrospect it seems that Medicare may have laid the foundation for the consensus on a desirable set of health insurance benefits which has apparently emerged in this country. Originally Medicare was proposed by successive Democratic administrations as a mandatory package of limited hospital care benefits. When a Republican counterproposal for voluntary health insurance was added to the bill, Congress enlarged the program to incorporate certain professional and other services and supplies used by the aged. Medicare benefits are both broad and deep. Most related medical services are included, either without limit as to quantity or with a high limit. In fact, extending a particular benefit without limits does not cost much beyond a certain point. It is a noteworthy advance in the public consensus concerning national health insurance policy when an identical benefit package is proposed for all population categories, as in the 1974 Nixon Administration bill. This is one necessary step toward curtailing, if not eliminating, a dual system of medical care.

It warrants recognition that not all the benefits that were offered under Medicare were promptly available. It took time and effort to organize home health services. Facilities for extended care did not then exist, and it is even questionable whether they exist today in skilled nursing homes, other than in name. There is reason to believe, too, that the general public misapprehended the extended-care benefit and that the ready availability of Medicaid as an alternative source of payment for long-term care served as a useful safety valve against widespread disappointment. With some allowance made for problems of transition, a broad and deep package of related benefits is, then, the second of the proposed criteria for assessing a national health insurance plan.

Single system of care

The shortness of the list of criteria so far—universality of enrollment and a broad and deep package of related benefits—is in part attributable to the exclusionary argument followed earlier to divert the pursuit of certain goals or objectives to other instrumentalities. However, I incline to a small number of criteria for appraising national health insurance plans for another reason. Although a long list of criteria can facilitate the building of a broad coalition in support of a program, only a short list can yield measures of trade-off terms between the several objectives that might lend themselves to comparison by ranking or weighing. If some sense of the quantitative values of the trade-off terms is important, a long list of criteria lacks credibility.

I have already hinted at a third criterion, namely, the compatibility of a particular health insurance plan with a single system of medical care for the well-to-do and the poor alike. This criterion is a matter of ultimate value judgment, in my opinion, and is not susceptible to the usual canons of proof through evidence. It has been suggested that even the scientific aspect of medical care may not always be the best possible in the medical school setting, where the poor receive care because attending staff and residents combine to search for the rare and subtle manifestations of disease. A case can be made perhaps that patients who feel inconvenience, discomfort, or possibly discriminated against are not so responsive to a prescribed regimen as they might be. I have no reluctance, however, to rest this criterion on the self-evident desirability of equity.

In the quest for a single system of care, a uniform package of benefits is necessary. Differences in fees according to source of payment, such as those adopted under Medicaid, are unacceptable. Other factors, including the organization of care and the behavioral characteristics of the population, are perhaps even more important for achieving a single system of care for all. Therefore, I am inclined to regard this goal as a longer-range target, rather than as an immediate requirement for a national health insurance plan. The target should remain visible, to be always more closely approached, rather than to be allowed to recede.

Provisions for provider reimbursement

I turn now to the financing of national health insurance. Does financing yield one or more additional criteria? If everybody is to be enrolled and the package of benefits is sizable, not everybody will be able to pay for it out of his own resources. This conclusion is incontrovertible. What is at issue is whether the amount of the health insurance premium will be linked to the particular individual with a determination of the public subsidy required to be made in each case, or whether the level of premium will merely be an actuarial average, with sources of payment determined for the entire health insurance fund. Although the latter would be far simpler, it might raise questions about the distribution of the tax burden, which are always controversial in this society and are seldom resolved satisfactorily. As a practical matter, in order to facilitate the passage of a national health insurance plan, it may be wise to dissociate provisions concerning the sources of financing from the other aspects of the plan. My point is obviously not that financing is to be omitted from a national health insurance plan but rather that I am disposed to be tolerant toward, and choose among, a fairly wide range of alternatives. The issues, arguments, and decisions on sources of financing are essentially political—both in the sense of ultimate value judgments and in the sense of the distribution of power. I propose that at this time sources of financing need not yield a criterion for assessing a national health insurance plan.

Closely related, but separable, is the issue of the patient's participation in financing through cost sharing at the time of illness. Briefly, the bases for advocating cost sharing are three-fold. One, cost sharing serves as a deterrent to the use of services and possibly as an incentive to shop around for services at a lower price. Two, it serves as a means to reduce the amount of insurance premium. Three, it serves to reserve general tax revenues for those public expenditure purposes which only such taxes can pay for, such as national defense or cash transfers.

It is unfortunate that the empirical literature to date on cost sharing is still so modest. It has been reported in a careful study at one site that co-insurance leads to a reduction in physician use and that the lowest socio-economic classes may incur the largest reduction in services. It is suggested by experience elsewhere that such reductions may not last. The first of these findings, namely that there is a large reduction in use associated with co-insurance, is the one that can be asserted with the most confidence at this time. If not eroded by the passage of time, the effect of co-insurance on the use of physician services is sizable. If we mean to overcome, or at least mitigate, the tendency of insurance to promote the use of services due to the lower out-of-pocket net price that the patient faces at the time of illness, then some cost sharing must take place.

In practice that has not occurred under Medicare, and it is not likely to occur under national health insurance. Rather, the policy is to permit the purchase of supplementary insurance to defray the amount of cost sharing. When the consumer is poor, cost sharing is often assumed by Medicaid or is occasionally waived by the provider of services. I am impelled to conclude that deterrence of use is not meant seriously as an argument in favor of cost sharing. If it were so intended, however, income relatedness would become important. It is reasonable to suppose that a given price or amount of cost sharing imposes greater weight upon a person with low income than on a person with high income.

Several economists have concerned themselves with the implications of health insurance for utilization and with the effects of cost sharing. None, however, has considered the practical implications of the policy to permit the purchase of supplementary insurance to defray the cost of cost sharing. Nor is there agreement on what is a proper measure of income in the context of illness, in view of the possibility of sizable fluctuations and permanent changes in income subsequent to the onset of major illness, as well as uncertainty about the future level of medical care expenditures. How will people learn of a change in their health insurance and copayment status with respect to income? How will they cope with such a change administratively? If the change, or notification about it, is retrospective, to what extent will it influence responses to price variation? How are we to avoid the so-called notch effect, whereby a consumer loses benefits when his income increases? Income related features also require a determination of the types of income to be assisted. In such a determination, is income in kind to be counted? In a given place, what is the point at which assistance from cost sharing ceases?

In light of the scarcity of empirical work on this topic, it seems incumbent upon one to be receptive to new evidence as it develops and to continue to be open to persuasion. Much about the administrative complexities inherent to an income-related cost-sharing scheme remains to be learned from experience. I believe that evaluation of experience in a large geographic area, like a state, can yield more useful knowledge than can analysis of the findings of a designed experiment in which several thousand families selected at random at three or four sites participate. The advantages of studying a large population in a contiguous area are the inclusion of possible responses on the supply side, acknowledgement of some of the emulative aspects of consumer behavior, and the greater stability of large numbers.

The second basis for advocating cost sharing is to keep down the level of premium. This consideration is obviously important in selling voluntary health insurance. Cost sharing under major medical insurance is readily understandable on the basis of this feature. It has always seemed to me that, if health insurance became mandatory, the level of premium could be determined by the size of the benefits package alone. Thus I am unable to understand the reason for cost sharing by the aged under Medicare. My understanding is not enhanced by recognition of the fact that many aged persons (approximately one-half) possess supplementary private insurance; another 10 percent are protected by Medicaid; and still others are not charged by their physicians for the co-insurance factor of 20 percent. Upon reflection, however, it is evident that even under mandatory enrollment, relying for financing on employer-employee contributions to premiums makes a lower premium desirable. Once the uniform benefits package is made broad and deep, it becomes necessary to supplement the insurance premium with private cost-sharing. In the context of financing through employer contributions, income relatedness is not pertinent.

The third basis of the rationale for cost sharing seems persuasive at a time of perpetual tightness in the federal budget. If we keep down the burden on the public fisc, not only can other things get done, which only the public fisc can pay for, but also the health services sector may enjoy greater latitude in spending. Certainly, the Social Security Trust Funds, which are usually treated as if they were quasi-private funds, have received authorized increases in benefits quite readily—much more so than they would have under regularly financed public programs. Ultimately, the decisive consideration may prove to be the balance between this factor—the desire to keep down the burden on the treasury—and administrative feasibility. If, in practice, cost-sharing payments turn out to be defaulted, they will have to be abandoned.

In summary, the rationale of cost sharing as a deterrent to use is not logically compatible with permitting the purchase of supplementary insurance to pay for cost sharing. Income relatedness would enter here, but not when cost sharing is intended to supplement employer contributions to premiums. Cost sharing for the purpose of saving tax funds for other public purposes is a new argument which must withstand the test of application and experience. It should be added that a policy decision adverse to substantial cost sharing need not preclude small copayments for extra services, such as night calls.

At this time I am not disposed to take a stand on cost sharing as a criterion for appraising a national health insurance plan. Too much remains to be learned about how it works and what its effects are. A sound policy to adopt is one that is reversible at a low or moderate cost.

It is, nevertheless, useful to note the importance of nonfinancial factors in influencing the use of health services. There is the physician-hospital relationship previously alluded to. Not to be overlooked is the sought-for patient-physician relationship, one of mutual confidence and trust. Of course, the fiduciary role of the professional in which he acts in behalf of the patient as if the latter's interests were his own, is not confined to medicine. These factors are, however, highly important in medicine. Financial incentives are not necessarily best adapted to the fostering of such a relationship, one of mutual trust and voluntary delegation of decision-making to the other party.

Preventive services pose a problem here, if their efficacy is granted. With or without insurance supplementation and with or without income relatedness, cost sharing should not apply to specified preventive services, such as maternal and infant care or well child care. For young families such payments are likely to be burdensome, even if they could be met in installments. It might be argued that such services are schedulable and can be planned for, so that they are not truly insurable risks. The controversy between health insurance and prepayment is an old one, however, and has not proved to be particularly fruitful. Perhaps more important, the number of personal health services that are currently presumed to be effective as preventive measures is quite small.

In the absence of cost sharing there would be no need to set a maximum limit on an individual's or family's expenditures for medical care. In the presence of cost sharing, it is necessary to set such a limit. It is worth noting that any computation of maximum liability on the part of the patient—individual or family—is bound to be an understatement to the extent that it omits the contribution to the insurance premium, excludes payments on covered benefits in excess of the stated fee, and, of course, excludes expenditure on items that are not among the covered benefits.

So far the discussion of financing has not yielded any criteria for assessing national health insurance plans which I am prepared to propose in light of existing knowledge. Appropriate provisions for reimbursement mechanisms and formulas are, however, a fourth criterion for assessing a national health insurance plan, in my judgment. I am aware that other students of the post-1965 rise in costs and expenditures do not attach as much importance to the influence of reimbursement as I do. Nevertheless, there is a widespread consensus that retrospective cost reimbursement of hospitals, which has been the major method for paying hospitals since 1965, must be ended. Since I can see no practical way to pay hospitals at uniform rates for a given service, it will be necessary to devise and adopt payment formulas that yield a fixed rate to individual hospitals for the period ahead. A fair summary of experience to date is that automatic reimbursement formulas do not work and that usually negotiations between provider and third-party payers are necessary. The several sources of payment acting separately are ineffective at controlling cost. It will be necessary to bring all major sources of payment together in negotiating both reimbursement formulas and amounts with individual institutions. In this country, experience with negotiated rates in behalf of all major sources of payment is lacking. The diverse and extensive experience of the several Canadian provinces in paying for hospital care since 1958 should be examined with care.

Regulatory mechanisms. Beyond the development of formulas and appropriate data sets lies the organization of effective regulatory mechanisms. The administrative problems of operating a national health insurance plan to cover a good part of an industry that is now spending more than $100 billion a year cannot be overestimated. There is bound to be a struggle for control by levels of government, between the private and public sectors, and between institutions and individuals. Personally, I should be inclined to look hard at the evidence on past performance as an indicator of future potentialities for contributing to this awesome task. Congressional hearings are highly useful for eliciting this type of information. Yet, it is doubtful that Congressional hearings can convey the atmosphere in which regulation actually takes place.

Speaking from personal knowledge, I must confess to a sense of disappointment over the extent to which the regulatory process in the health field seems to have taken on some of the adversary characteristics of criminal court proceedings. It is not only the consumer who is suing for malpractice today, but the provider is suing the health insurance plan plus the state regulatory agency, while the regulatory agency sues a health insurance plan plus its individual board members. Power and its exercise have displaced the ordinary civilities based on a comity of interests that usually accompany relationships between legitimate governors and the governed. Economists have traditionally tended to distrust regulation on the ground that the regulated tend to become the regulators. What has not been foreseen by proponents of regulation is the possible runaway nature of regulatory power when carried out with full discretion. As much as possible, discretionary authority must be limited, even as ministerial functions are extended, with both subject to the constraints of a free flow of information that is equally accessible to all. In a complex society such as ours, it is obviously not practical to dispense with regulation. But the time has come to recognize regulation's potential for caprice and willful instability. It is necessary to aim for responsible due process, uniformly applied, quite apart from the substantive results that we seek.

With respect to reimbursement for physician services, I am persuaded of two points. The prevailing method of payment under Medicare of customary and usual fees, subject to a prevailing cutoff, is inflationary per se. And permitting the nonacceptance of assignment of fees by the provider is both inflationary and conducive to a dual standard of care. Perhaps it is permissible to have two or three levels of practitioners with corresponding levels of fees; I do not know. It is certainly necessary to protect the patient fully against extra out-of-pocket costs and against provider discrimination, whether real or perceived.

Ease of compliance

A fifth criterion for appraising national health insurance plans is ease of compliance by the consumer. After all, it does not matter that the expert can read statutes and regulations only by working at it. The provider can pass on the extra expense of an expanded administrative staff. The bureaucracy always gets paid, but the patient does whatever he must do on his own time, at his own cost. It is important that he receive all the health insurance benefits that he is entitled to, that he be enabled to rely on continuing to receive them, and that he fully understand the consequences of his own misdeeds and those of others.

Health services are delivered locally. The choice of providers available to the consumer may be limited. Changing providers is a drastic remedy, perhaps too drastic to be applied routinely. Employing an independent, impartial ombudsman may be worthwhile.

Recently a health card has been proposed for every enrollee in the national health insurance plan. Under the plan no cash would flow between the patient and the participating provider. The health card plan would pay the provider both the insurance benefit and the amount of cost sharing—all the time having kept track of the status of the patient's deductible. The patient would reimburse the health card plan, being allowed to pay out his obligation in installments. The idea is appealingly simple. What we do not know is how well it would work, especially for people not accustomed to the use of credit cards. Nor is it clear what would be the consequences of failure to meet the payments due. It is important to acquire some experience in the use of a health card by diverse population groups and to ascertain the features that work and the features that are likely to prove troublesome.

The HMO Option

No discussion of national health policy can pass muster today without some reference to the HMO (Health Maintenance Organization). At the outset, it must be said that some of the discriminatory practices formerly employed against prepaid group practice organizations have no basis in objective fact, do not serve the public interest, and should cease throughout the land. To provide an HMO option, where practicable, under national health insurance is only fair play and in accord with the notion that free choice is a basic value in our society.

Some students of the health services would go further and favor the promotion of the HMO on the grounds that it would yield appreciable savings, particularly in hospital use, and that by virtue of its pro-competitive characteristics the HMO would serve to reduce the purview of public intervention through planning and regulation. Their central assumption is that the consumer can learn enough about the quality of medical care to recognize it and to choose gradations in quality on the basis of price. Indeed, it is argued, if the consumer could and would act on such information, his interests would be identical with those of the provider and of the prepayment plan.

Elsewhere I have raised a number of questions about these assumptions concerning the HMO and the expectations they raise. The fact is that information about quality of care, particularly in the ambulatory setting, is not available. The reported savings in hospital use by subscribers to one form of the HMO, prepaid group practice, are confounded by the presence of a tight or inaccessible bed supply. Prepaid group practice has not manifested extra productivity in the use of personnel.

It may well be that its proponents have oversold the HMO and thereby done it an injustice. Under voluntary health insurance a package of benefits that is too broad cannot be marketed. It does not do the HMO any good to have a broad package prescribed for it. It does not do the HMO any good to be subjected to quality controls that apply to nobody else. There is no known way today to standardize HMO and other populations with respect to medical care premiums. Laws requiring certificates of need may be in conflict with the unique local requirements of the HMO. The principal point here is that the problems of the HMO are sufficiently specialized to warrant separate attention. For the purposes of a national health insurance plan, it suffices to offer the HMO option without favor and without prejudice.

Summary

Let me summarize. I have essayed to draw on our record of experience under prepayment, and this record reflects many accomplishments as well as failures. I emphasize conserving the financial mechanism for those purposes that it is best designed to serve. I avoid taking a strong stand on issues on which sound evidence is lacking. Accordingly, at this time, I propose the following five criteria for assessing a national health insurance plan: (1) universal enrollment; (2) a uniform package of benefits, both broad and deep, for all; (3) furtherance of the goal of a single system of medical care for all (or at least not promoting any incentives toward the opposite direction); (4) effective provision for provider reimbursement, with a responsible and responsive exercise of regulatory authority rooted in a free flow of information; and (5) ease of compliance by consumers, with attention to the validation of their expectations from the insurance plan. I believe that this modest list of criteria is both moderate and attainable.

PREVIOUS VOLUMES IN THIS SERIES

The Future of Economic Policy, Myron H. Ross, Editor, 1966
Michigan Business Papers, No. 44, 1967

Paul W. McCracken	*The Political Position of the Council of Economic Advisers*
Robert Eisner	*Fiscal and Monetary Policy for Economic Growth*
Theodore W. Schultz	*Public Approaches to Minimize Poverty*
Jesse W. Markham	*Antitrust Policy after a Decade of Vigor*
Kenneth E. Boulding	*The Price System and the Price of the Great Society*
Robert Triffin	*International Monetary Reform*

Key Factors in Economic Growth, Raymond E. Zelder, Editor, 1967
Michigan Business Papers, No. 48, 1968

Martin Bronfenbrenner	*Japanese Economic Development in the Meiji Era, 1867-1912*
Nicholas Spulber	*Is the U.S.S.R. Going Capitalist?*
Milos Samardzija	*Economic Growth and Workers' Management in Yugoslavia*
Lauchlin Currie	*The Crisis in Latin American Development*
Edmundo Flores	*The Alliance for Progress and the Mexican Revolution*
Alexander Eckstein	*The Economic Development of Communist China*

The Cost of Conflict, John A. Copps, Editor, 1968
Michigan Business Papers, No. 51, 1969

Kenneth E. Boulding	*The Threat System*
Thomas C. Schelling	*The Diplomacy of Violence*
Seymour Melman	*The Price of Peace*
Murray L. Weidenbaum	*Towards a Peacetime Economy*
Roger E. Bolton	*National Defense and Regional Development*
Emile Benoit	*Economic Adjustments to Peace in the Far East and to Ending the Arms Race*

America's Cities, Wayland D. Gardner, Editor, 1969
Michigan Business Papers, No. 54, 1970

Wilbur R. Thompson	*The Process of Metropolitan Development: American Experience*
Hugh O. Nourse	*Industrial Location and Land Use in Metropolitan Areas*
Richard F. Muth	*The Economics of Slum Housing*
Dick Netzer	*Urban Government Finance and Urban Development*
Werner Z. Hirsch	*The Urban Challenge to Governments*

Antitrust Policy and Economic Welfare, Werner Sichel, Editor, 1970
Michigan Business Papers, No. 56, 1970

Walter Adams	*The Case for a Comprehensive and Vigorous Antitrust Policy*
Jules Backman	*Holding the Reins on the Trust Busters*
Almarin Phillips	*Antitrust Policies: Could They Be Tools of the Establishment?*
Richard B. Heflebower	*The Conglomerate in American Industry: A Special Antitrust Wrinkle*
Jesse W. Markham	*Structure versus Conduct Criteria in Antitrust*
William G. Shepherd	*Changing Contrasts in British and American Antitrust Policies*

Economic Policies in the 1970s, Alfred K. Ho, Editor, 1971
Michigan Business Papers, No. 57, 1971

James M. Buchanan	*Economists, the Government, and the Economy*
Martin Bronfenbrenner	*Nixonomics and Stagflation Reconsidered*
David I. Fand	*Some Observations on Current Stabilization Policy*
Gardner Ackley	*International Inflation*
Harry G. Johnson	*Inflation: A "Monetarist" View*
Bela Balassa	*Prospects and Problems of British Entry into the Common Market*

The Economics of Environmental Problems, Frank C. Emerson, Editor,
1972
Michigan Business Papers, No. 58, 1973

<table>
<tr><td>Joseph L. Fisher</td><td>*An Introduction to Environmental Economics*</td></tr>
<tr><td>Lester B. Lave</td><td>*The Economic Costs of Air Pollution*</td></tr>
<tr><td>Robert H. Haveman</td><td>*The Political Economy of Federal Water Quality Policy*</td></tr>
<tr><td>William S. Vickery</td><td>*The Economics of Congestion Control in Urban Transportation*</td></tr>
<tr><td>Jerome Rothenberg</td><td>*The Evaluation of Alternative Public Policy Approaches to Environmental Control*</td></tr>
</table>

The Economics of Education, Myron H. Ross, Editor, 1973
Michigan Business Papers, No. 59, 1974

<table>
<tr><td>Charles C. Killingsworth</td><td>*The Evaluation of Manpower Programs*</td></tr>
<tr><td>Samuel Bowles</td><td>*The Integration of Higher Education into the Wage-Labor System*</td></tr>
<tr><td>Richard Eckaus</td><td>*How Much and What Kinds of Education for Economic Development?*</td></tr>
<tr><td>Theodore W. Shultz</td><td>*Investments in Ourselves: Opportunities and Implications*</td></tr>
<tr><td>Jerry Miner</td><td>*Methods of Finance and the Organization and Administration of Local Schools*</td></tr>
</table>